East-West Healing

Integrating Chinese and Western Medicines for Optimal Health

MAY LOO, M.D.
AND
JACK MAGUIRE

John Wiley & Sons, Inc.
New York • Chichester • Weinheim • Brisbane • Singapore • Toronto

~ 3106 ~

Published by John Wiley & Sons, Inc.
Published simultaneously in Canada

Illustrations copyright © 2001 by Jackie Aher

Design and production by Navta Associates, Inc.

Grateful acknowledgment is made to Effie Chow, Ph.D., R.N., for permission to include the Chow Five-Element Meditation; and to North Atlantic Books for permission to include excerpts and food lists from *Healing with Whole Foods: Oriental Traditions and Modern Nutrition* by Paul Pitchford, copyright © 1993. Reprinted with permission of North Atlantic Books, Berkeley, California, USA.

This publication is designed to provide accurate and authoritative information in regard to the subject matter covered. It is sold with the understanding that the publisher is not engaged in rendering professional services. If professional advice or other expert assistance is required, the services of a competent professional person should be sought.

Library of Congress Cataloging-in-Publication Data

Loo, May
    East-West healing : integrating Chinese and Western medicines for
optimal health / May Loo and Jack Maguire
        p. cm.
    Includes bibliographical references.
    ISBN 0-471-35603-4 (cloth : alk. paper)
    1. Health. 2. Medicine, Chinese. 3. Healing. 4. Alternative medicine.
I. Maguire, Jack. II. Title.

RA776.5 .L66 2001
615.5'0951—dc21   00-068601

Printed in the United States of America

10 9 8 7 6 5 4 3 2 1

To my daughters,
Alyssa and Alexandra,
with Love

Acknowledgments

With thanks to the teachings of Dr. Effie Chow, Maciocia Giovanni, Dan Bensky, Dr. Joseph Helms, and Paul Pitchford, whose works I have used as references. With thanks to Tom Miller for his patience; thanks to Faith Hamlin, Sean McCormack, Ed Myers, Jack Maguire, Jackie Aher, and Andrew Ellis.

Thanks especially to my family for their love, understanding, and support.

Contents

(ADHD, ADD) • Baldness (or Hair Loss) • Bedwetting (Enuresis) •
Belching, Excessive • Bladder Infection (Urinary Cystitis) • Bleeding,
External • Bleeding, Internal • Bruises • Bulimia • Cold, Common
• Cold Sores (or Mouth Ulcers) • Colic • Conjunctivitis ("Pink Eye") •
Constipation • Cough • Diaper Rash • Diarrhea • Drooling • Ear
Infection • Ear-Ringing (Tinnitus) • Eczema • Edema (Swelling) •
Emotional Problems • Fatigue • Gastritis • Headache • Hemorrhoids
• Hiccups • Hives • Hypertension (High Blood Pressure) • Impetigo •
Insomnia (or Sleep Problems) • Jaundice, Newborn • Jet Lag • Menstrual
Problems • Motion Sickness • Nervous Stomach • Nosebleed (Epistaxis)
• Obesity • Pain • Scars • Seizure • Sighing, Excessive or Chronic •
Snoring • Sore Throat (Pharyngitis or Tonsillitis) • Stuttering • Thrush •
Toothache

Introduction

Western medicine is a technologically advanced healing system based on scientific principles and scientifically verified facts. It began in the seventeenth century and has occupied an authoritative position in health care worldwide ever since. However, it is not the only health care system that has proven its worth or that is utilized worldwide. Nor has it shown itself capable of resolving—or, in many cases, even addressing—the full range of health problems that people experience.

Today more and more people are combining Western medicine with another kind of medicine that offers a perfect complement: Chinese medicine. It's a time-tested and highly effective therapeutic system based not only on a profound philosophy of our vital connection with the natural world, but also on a rich tradition of healing experiences and knowledge.

Chinese medicine has successfully treated human health problems for thousands of years. Westerners only started learning about this system in the 1600s, however, when Jesuits returned to Europe after travels in China and told stories of "healing with needles," or acupuncture—just one technique among many in the Chinese arsenal. Because of language barriers, translations of Chinese medical texts into European languages didn't appear until the twentieth century. Only following President Nixon's historic trip to China in 1972 did this grand medical tradition enter the consciousness of the mainstream American public.

The past decade has brought a surge of interest in Chinese medicine among Westerners. This interest has occurred for several reasons:

- The skyrocketing expense of professional Western medical care is inspiring more and more people to take a personal initiative in preventing and treating illness. Chinese medicine offers simple, low-, or no-cost methods we can easily use to care for ourselves and our loved ones.
- The incidence of complicated, stress-related medical problems such as heart disease, immune deficiency problems, allergies, and musculoskeletal pain continues to increase dramatically each year. These and other similar illnesses respond especially well to Chinese medicine's combined attention to body, mind, and spirit.
- A growing regard for environmental health and the natural processes of life prompts us to seek a more natural means of health care, which Chinese medicine furnishes.
- Greater contact with Chinese culture is generating new respect among Westerners, including doctors and scientists, for Chinese medicine. We see this respect, for example, in media reports on the success of acupuncture in treating addiction, of Qigong and Tai Chi in maintaining healthy blood pressure and physical mobility, and of Chinese dietary practices in bolstering the immune system.

This book enables you to have the best of both worlds of health care: East and West. Drawing on my twenty-year career as a doctor, researcher, and teacher in both areas of medicine, it offers the following advantages:

- It clearly explains the basic principles of Chinese and Western medical care and how they function in determining our well-being, including the concept of Qi—the life energy circulating throughout our bodies.
- It illuminates and validates these concepts by relating them to Western ones and to real-life examples of healing.
- It shows you how to perform key Chinese health practices that are easy, safe, and effective, especially in combination with Western ones. Among them are acupressure (pressing major healing points on the body), basic dietary guidelines, physical exercises, and meditation and breathing activities.
- It reveals healthier ways to eat and drink, based on centuries of Chinese medical experience, including how to select and prepare common foods and beverages.
- It offers physical exercises that adults or children can comfortably do in minutes a day to feel more alive and to ensure their ongoing health.
- It equips readers to conduct more thorough and useful health evaluations of themselves and others—both before and after symptoms of illness appear.

The heart of the book, chapter 6, is a concise, practical, easy-reference home guide to treating more than fifty common health problems using both Chinese and Western medical practices. The entries cover specific physical illnesses and symptoms as well as illness-prone conditions (such as alcoholism or smoking) and emotional complaints (such as anger or depression). Other sections of the book supply information about herbs and guidelines for using Chinese medicine to counteract the side effects of Western medications.

In addition to helping you work with qualified professionals, the book will hopefully motivate you to explore other Chinese medical practices, such as herbal therapy and acupuncture. The relatively simpler, more convenient treatments recommended in these pages were chosen to facilitate safe, practical personal and home health care by nonprofessionals in any kind of living environment. Tapping into more complex procedures such as herbal therapy or acupuncture can give you even more comprehensive care for many of the conditions addressed in this book, as well as treatments for healing more complicated conditions.

Above all, this book is designed to demystify Chinese medicine, to make its virtues more apparent, compelling, and accessible to you, and to help you integrate it with Western medical care in the easiest, most comfortable, and most effective ways possible. At first, Chinese medical terminology—which consists mostly of plain, commonly used words—can sound paradoxically strange to Westerners, who are accustomed to associating health care with technical jargon. Nevertheless, Chinese medical terminology quickly becomes familiar and sensible as you read more about it; this familiarity occurs partly because of Chinese medicine's foundation in Nature and partly because of the many inherent, easily grasped correspondences that exist between Chinese and Western health concepts.

For example, the five principal causes of disease are categorized by the Chinese as Wind, Heat, Cold, Humidity, and Dryness. According to these categories, a common cold has long been classified as an attack of Wind Cold, mainly because it has always been known that people can become sick when they are exposed to wind and cold. Western microbiology now tells us that viruses causing the common cold are airborne and, therefore, can be "carried" in a cold wind.

More points of connection between Chinese and Western concepts will be clarified in these pages as appropriate. A glossary in the back of the book gives you an accessible, central reference source to use for checking the meaning and correspondences relating to individual Chinese words or expressions.

The final power and responsibility for maintaining our own health and that of our families rests in ourselves—in the day-to-day ways in which we eat, move, sleep, interact, and handle physical, emotional, and spiritual challenges. By gently keeping us in harmony with human nature and the natural world as we go through our days, Chinese medicine picks up where Western medicine leaves off.

The goal of this book is to help you integrate both of these great medical traditions into your home life in the manner that best suits you. Besides giving you more skill and success in treating common health complaints, the procedures it describes will help you understand yourself better and bring you closer to those you love. May you use it in good health!

PART I

The Basics
of East-West
Medicine

CHAPTER 1

Understanding East-West Healing

Western science has brought us many medical miracles, from aspirin to zooplasty (transferring tissue from other animals to human beings). Despite these technological marvels, however, we seem to need something more to stay healthy.

The truth is that along with the miracles of Western science has come an increasingly stressful and unwholesome way of life, fueled by a haphazard diet of processed foods and aggravated by a wide range of poorly understood biological and technological hazards. We and our loved ones often get sick with vague but real illnesses that we don't know how to treat. And we worry about relying solely on drugs, money, and our own sense of powerlessness to take care of ourselves and our families. Despite the many marvels that Western medicine can offer, it clearly lacks an essential element that can help us lead healthier lives and cope better with illnesses at home.

More and more people find this missing element in Chinese medicine. This rich, nature-based tradition consistently addresses a person's entire being—physical, mental, emotional, and spiritual—in the context of his or her day-to-day lifestyle. In doing so, it serves as the perfect companion to Western medical science, which tends to focus more technically on the particulars of a specific illness or condition.

As a doctor trained in both Western and Chinese medicine, I've found that combining the two systems provides the finest, most thorough, and most humane health care possible. Here are a few examples from my practice:

- Sally suffered from severe migraine headaches. She took two oral medications regularly to keep them at bay and a third drug when the pain grew unbearable. Unfortunately, two of the medications were hazardous during pregnancy, and she and her new husband longed to start a family.

  I taught both Sally and her husband a routine of pressing key points on Sally's body, based on the Chinese medical practice of acupressure, to help prevent or alleviate her migraines. Sally also learned a special style of breathing, advocated in Chinese medicine, to relax herself physically and emotionally. Over a few months, she was able to taper off using the two risky drugs for good; in their place, Sally started taking the third, more benign medication for quick relief of her occasional headaches. Now she and her husband have a healthy newborn son.

- Two-year-old Melissa had frequent ear infections since she was six months old. She usually needed several courses of antibiotics each time she had an acute infection, followed by a daily maintenance antibiotic for months afterward. The medicine caused diarrhea and diaper rash. Jan, her mother, suspected that Melissa's four-year-old brother was bringing germs home from preschool, but she hated to withdraw him from his program.

Instead, I showed Jan special massages derived from Chinese medicine that she could give Melissa *and* her brother to bolster their immunity. I also advised Jan how to make simple shifts in their diet, according to Chinese medical principles, even before they showed signs of congestion. And I talked to her about how to combine these practices with commonsense Western home medical care. Now both kids are healthier than before. When Melissa does get an earache, she needs much less Western medication, and Jan can follow other Chinese-based massage and dietary guidelines to reduce any unwanted side effects of the medication.

- David works long hours at a start-up company. A few months ago he was caught up in a vicious cycle of drinking ten to twelve cups of coffee a day to help him stay awake, and then taking sleeping pills at night for insomnia. After a full day's work and dinner at home, he usually felt too exhausted to do anything but collapse in front of the TV. It bothered him *and* his family that he wasn't up to more interaction, but there didn't seem to be much he could do about it. He tried for weeks to cut down his daily coffee intake and went to bed earlier to try to get more sleep without taking pills. He was only mildly successful, but he felt more tired during the day without his coffee and still couldn't really shake his evening sluggishness.

  Then I showed David how to increase his energy with a little self-administered acupressure and a few simple exercises. He could do these in his chair at the office or almost anywhere else he found himself with a few moments to spare. Within two weeks of self-administering this program, he began to feel much more energetic and communicative in the evenings. Although he still needs one or two cups of coffee each day to feel human—and, occasionally, a sleeping pill on a bad night—the program has resolved the crisis. It's now second nature for him to do the acupressure and exercises, and both he and his family are reaping the benefits.

These examples suggest only a fraction of the ways in which Chinese medicine can complement its Western counterpart to treat health problems more successfully. In addition, Chinese practices can work wonderfully on their own to help keep the mind, body, and spirit in good, well-balanced shape so that health problems don't arise in the first place—or, if they do, so that they are less severe than they otherwise might have been.

Western medicine relies heavily on physician-based care, laboratory tests, and prescription drugs. One of the beauties of Chinese medical treatment is that so much of it consists of easy procedures that anyone can follow comfortably and confidently. All of the practices I recommend in the book—acupressure, dietary modification, stress management, proper breathing, meditation, and exercise—fall into this category. You don't need any special equipment, skill, or training to apply them in caring for yourself or your loved ones.

Two Opinions Are Better Than One

The core difference between Western and Chinese medicine lies in their concept of the human body. The two traditions take two different approaches. It isn't that one approach is false and the other is true. Instead, each offers a different perspective that has its own validity and its own limitations. When we combine the two approaches in our personal and family health care, we can get the best of both worlds.

Most of you are likely to be far more familiar with the Western perspective than the Chinese one, since you have grown up in a Western culture and have always relied on Western forms of health care. With this in mind, here and elsewhere in the book I will often describe Chinese medical principles and features in more detail than Western ones. Right now I'll establish the most basic differences between them.

Western medicine approaches the human body from an anatomic and biochemical standpoint. It sees us as physical beings made of many parts that can be dissected down to tiny, independent components. Western medicine adopts the philosophy that we are unique beings and that our intellect places us as far superior to all other living things. Chinese medicine approaches the human body from an energetic and functional standpoint. It sees us as whole beings made of energetic, physical, emotional, and spiritual parts that are intimately related. Chinese medicine adopts the philosophy that Man is a miniature replica of Nature, a living entity of Nature no more superior than the lion or even the tree.

Chinese medicine examines the life and health of a human being from a broader field of reference, one that includes forces and relationships that are not so easy to isolate or see. The guidelines in this book derive from four key concepts in Chinese medical theory:

1. the existence of Qi or a field of "vital energy" coursing throughout the body
2. the principle of Yin-Yang or "dynamic opposites" in the way the body functions
3. the link to Nature through the Five Elements—Water, Wood, Fire, Earth, and Metal—in human existence
4. the constant interconnection of the Mind, Body, and Spirit in human health

I am calling these four items "concepts" for the sake of convenience, just as I might apply the label "concept" to the principle of cause and effect or to the theory of bacterial infection. Calling them concepts doesn't mean that they have no factual foundation. In reality, the truth of these concepts has been verified by centuries of expert Chinese medical research and treatment. Even Western science, after a relatively short period of time spent investigating Chinese medicine, is beginning to validate on its own terms certain portions of these four concepts—a subject I discuss more specifically (when it's appropriate) throughout the rest of the book.

Nor do I mean to suggest that these four concepts operate in isolation from one another. During each moment of a human being's existence, they all function simultaneously and interdependently to keep that person alive and healthy, and any problem affecting one influences the other three. For the purpose of learning more about these four concepts, however, let's look at each one separately.

Qi: Our Vital Energy

Qi (pronounced CHEE) can be roughly translated into English as "vital energy." In its broadest sense, Qi refers to the natural energy that permeates all life forms and connects them with one another in what we call the natural world. Thus any personal illness can be said to relate intimately to the natural environment surrounding the person—including other people, the climate, the land, the air, and so on.

On the more individual level, Qi refers to the flow or field of energy within each human being. Thus illness can be said to result from internal Qi problems that manifest themselves in an individual's body, mind, and behavior.

This concept of Qi represents the primary distinction between Chinese and Western medical theory. As I indicated above, the latter tradition is based on scientific principles of physiology and chemistry rather than on the more broad-based principle of energy. Science has uncovered and continues to add tremendous amounts of information to our understanding of the biophysical and biochemical nature of the human being,

14

down to subcellular levels. This information is concretely evident—something that can be seen, measured, and quantified.

On the other hand, Qi, the bioenergetic basis of Chinese medicine, cannot yet be directly seen, measured, or quantified. It manifests itself only in the varying degrees of a person's health or illness. I'm confident that technological advances within the near future will enable us to perceive Qi more directly. It's already being determined, for example, that Qi has electromagnetic properties. Qi is also starting to be described as the wave or energy part of the human body, while the anatomical-biochemical model is the particle or matter part. Meanwhile, a new field of bioenergetic medicine is emerging in the West that is making giant strides toward interweaving the two traditions.

So where in the human body *is* this Qi, this energy that can't be seen directly? Chinese medicine has established over the centuries that Qi is everywhere in the body. It circulates in the body along channels called meridians. As part of the blood, it moves within blood vessels. As part of organs and tissues, it functions within them. It is the foundation of our being.

Throughout its system of channels, Qi flows steadily in one direction. When our Qi flow is balanced and uninterrupted, we are healthy. When it's unbalanced or blocked, we become ill. Everything we do and everything around us can affect our Qi: our diet, our emotions, our thoughts, our actions and interactions, our lifestyles, and our environment.

In Chinese medicine, the three building blocks of life are Qi, blood, and fluid—a fact that will become more clear as I discuss individual health situations later in the book. This system correlates roughly in Western medicine to the body's network of blood, fluid, and nerves. While many acupuncture points are found along nerve routes, Qi meridians do not follow nerve patterns, and the nervous system is not defined in Chinese medicine.

In a moment I'll give more specifics about how Qi flows and functions within the human body. I'll also return to the topic again and again throughout the book as it relates to understanding and treating particular illnesses and conditions. Right now let's look at the larger picture: how Qi in general is influenced by—and manifests itself in—every aspect of an individual's life. Imagine a fairly typical, thirty-five-year-old American woman we'll call Sandra: a hardworking computer company manager with an equally hardworking husband, Tom, and a four-year-old son, Chad. Let's put ourselves in her shoes for a while.

A Day in the Life of Qi

Sandra has a frantic afternoon at work on Thursday. She dashes out of her office at 5:45 P.M., leaving piles of unfinished papers on her desk, so she can pick up Chad before his day care center closes at six. She curses the traffic and pounds on the steering wheel as she waits for the last red light to turn. Chad is waiting anxiously with his jacket on (it's a chilly, late-winter evening) when she finally arrives at the day care center.

Happy to see his mother after waiting so long, Chad begins blurting out all the exciting things that happened in day care: he dropped his sandwich in the sandbox, the rabbit got out of the cage, Stephanie fell, and so on. Sandra can only half listen, preoccupied as she is with thoughts about dinner, bills, housecleaning chores, and that unfinished pile of papers on her desk.

Sensing her distraction, Chad pulls out his video game and starts pressing buttons, while Sandra pulls up at a drive-in ATM to get some cash for a fast-food dinner. The two of them are chewing their last morsels of burger and sipping their last drops of cold juice as they pull into the driveway at home.

The next order of business is getting Chad to take a bath. After bathing (and, against her good intentions, yelling at) a squirming Chad, Sandra parks him in front of the TV. Then Tom comes home, also exhausted, and pops the leftover bag of fast food into the microwave for his dinner. They talk about bills as he washes down his burger with a cold beer. Afterward Tom plays with Chad until it's time to put him to bed.

"Better give Chad some more decongestant," Sandra calls out to Tom while taking a sleeping pill herself.

Two weeks later, Sandra goes to see her doctor with complaints about general fatigue and irritability. Her physical examination turns out normal, as do all her laboratory tests. The diagnosis is "psychosomatic symptoms secondary to stress; mild depression." She refuses the prescription for antidepressants but takes the refill for sleeping pills.

At the same time, Chad has to see the pediatrician. His cold has lingered, and now he also has a sore throat. Sandra mentions to the doctor that Chad seems to be having more temper tantrums. After prescribing medication for the sore throat, the doctor assures her that the frequency of tantrums she describes lies within the normal range for a child Chad's age, which means there is no need for lab tests.

Among other things, this minisaga of Sandra and Chad (excluding Tom for simplicity's sake) points out the differences between Western medicine and Chinese medicine. In Western medicine, a physical examination or lab test that turns out "normal" means the person is considered to have normal health that needs no treatment. According to studies, as many as 95 percent of people who experience vague physical complaints are told by their doctors, "Nothing is wrong." From the standpoint of Western medicine, that's true. From the Chinese perspective, however, the truth lies much deeper.

Unhealthy changes occur in a person's energetic or Qi system long before any physical signs or abnormal lab results can be detected. Those few hours Thursday night for Sandra and Chad were loaded with adverse influences on their Qi. A basic knowledge of Chinese medicine would have made Sandra more aware of those influences and more equipped to modify, counteract, or eliminate them before they finally produced tangible symptoms.

For example, Chinese medicine emphasizes that healthy Qi flow corresponds to the natural order and rhythm of the universe. During the day, it is active; during the evening, it is winding down for overnight rest. On that busy Thursday evening, Sandra was physically, mentally, and emotionally very agitated. Everything she put herself through was as unnatural for her body as making a hibernating bear dance in the snow.

Chad, too, was much more active than was beneficial. The last thing he needed at 6:00 P.M. was a video game designed to make the brain react continuously on a split-second basis. Nor did he need his mother to yell at him, even if only a couple of times in the heat of the moment, for doing things that most four-year-olds do. The result of all these factors was Qi stagnation and deficiency—a state that can ultimately lead to the development of physical, emotional, and behavioral problems.

Another Thursday night event that was bound to have a negative impact on the Qi of all three individuals in many different ways was the fast-food dinner—both the food items themselves (among other things, loaded with artificial additives) and the quick, distracted manner in which they were eaten. Chapter 4 will go into this issue in more detail, giving you a sense of the problems involved in that kind of dinner. For the moment, let me give you one small insight into the matter.

Remember the cold juice Sandra and Chad drank (not to mention Tom's cold beer)? That coldness alone can create Qi problems. Western medicine tells us that whenever our bodies get cold, our metabolism slows down. So think what happens to Qi flow when we drink cold drinks with our meals. That's right: the frigidity shocks our digestive system's Qi and impedes its performance when it should be working its best. Since nutrition is crucial to our overall Qi balance, when the digestive Qi is impaired, our whole body will eventually also be affected.

And that's not the only potential problem with Sandra's and Chad's beverages. According to Chinese medicine, foods and drinks contain healing properties relative to their own natural coolness or warmth, which, in turn, depends on their season of harvest, as we'll discuss in chapter 4. There's a natural reason to eat, for instance, more fruit in the summer than in the winter. When we follow this pattern, we work in harmony with nature to maintain good health.

Nowadays, thanks to freezing and preservatives, we can eat fruit all year long, which can disrupt the healthy, seasonal rhythms of our bodies. The solution is not to eliminate eating fruit in the winter, but to avoid overdoing it, and, in general, to be more mindful about eating in tune with the time of year. Just as your body adjusts itself to suit the season, so should your diet.

Finally, the story of Sandra and Chad's Thursday evening discloses a host of technological interferences with their natural Qi. The sad truth is that these interferences are facts of life for anyone living in the industrialized world.

The most fundamental one is the alteration of natural day-night patterns caused by artificial lighting, which leads us to engage in all sorts of activities that are unhealthy for the particular time period involved. Then there's the issue of Sandra's almost total reliance on chemical medications to give her own and her child's health problems a quick fix. It's an understandable pattern of behavior for anyone living in the West, where science has long been the highest—if not the only—authority in health care. But for all the symptomatic relief that sleeping pills, decongestants, antacids, or antibiotics may bring us, they also can trigger serious Qi disturbances. Some are indirectly acknowledged through side-effect warnings on labels, such as gastrointestinal symptoms. Others are unmentioned and, to Western science at least, unclassifiable, such as a feeling of heaviness after taking a medication. That doesn't mean they aren't real or won't eventually result in vary palpable illness.

Another technological threat to Sandy and Chad's health on that Thursday was the electromagnetic bombardment of their bodies by all the gadgetry surrounding them, including Sandra's computer, Chad's video games, the microwave and TV in their home, and even the car itself, a moving electromagnetic field. This kind of bombardment almost certainly compromises Qi performance and, as citizens of the Western world, we all experience a heavy dose of it daily. We may not be able to escape it entirely, but we can at least become more aware of it and do what we reasonably can to reduce its negative effects. Chinese medicine can help enormously in this effort.

Qi Channels and Organ Systems

As you read through and use this book, you'll learn more about the different Qi channels that function in the body and how to help them operate to the best of their ability. These channels are roughly analogous to the organ systems in Western medicine, but there's a key distinction.

Organ systems in Western medicine indicate concrete *physical* entities. The lung system, for example, refers to the physical organs in the chest cavity and their immediately supporting physical structures. In Chinese medicine, organ-related Qi systems are *functional* entities that go beyond any one specific physical site in the body. For example, Lung Qi (Chinese-related terms are capitalized for easy reference) moves through a channel that goes to the chest, but also has points down the inside of the arm to the fingertips—points that can be manipulated to influence Lung Qi functioning.

In a way, you can think of the Qi system as an "energetically extended" organ system. To appreciate this interpretation, let's compare the Western and the Chinese definitions of an organ system.

Strictly speaking, a Western organ system has a specific network of blood vessels and nerves that connect it with other parts of the body. Think of the lungs, for example. They're supplied by pulmonary blood vessels and nerves that are connected with other blood vessels and nerves in the body. Thus a blood sample taken from the wrist or the groin can reflect oxygen activity in the lung.

The Qi system in Chinese medicine also connects organs with other parts of the body, but in a somewhat different manner. For example, the Lung Qi meridian goes to the lung and also down the front of the arm, and connects to other Qi channels. While Western medicine uses accessible areas along the bloodstream to get biochemical information about lung activity, Chinese medicine stimulates various spots along a Lung Qi meridian (known as acupressure points or acupuncture points) to bring about healthy Qi activity in that system. This book shows you how to stimulate appropriate acupressure spots manually to alleviate a wide range of common health problems.

To find out specifically where these points and others are located, see the diagrams in appendix D.

Yin-Yang Balance: Our Dynamic Nature

Both Chinese medicine and Western medicine aim toward achieving a healthy state of balance within the body. Western medicine calls this state homeostasis. Chinese medicine calls it Yin-Yang balance. The two words symbolize opposing qualities that exist both in the nature of the universe and in each person's individual nature, such as night and day, cold and hot, female and male, deficiency and excess.

To call these pairs opposites does not mean that they can't coexist at the same time. The Yin-Yang principle tells us that opposites are in constant evolution toward each other and that there is a component of one in the other. Within Yin there is

Yang and within Yang there is Yin. The dynamism between the opposites is what keeps all of Nature in equilibrium instead of chaos.

It can be difficult for Westerners to grasp this principle because Aristotelian logic has trained us to believe that opposites are mutually exclusive: either a table is square or it's circular—it cannot be both. Actually, from a Chinese perspective it *can* be both, if you look beyond what is obvious and see the continuum of change that connects the two. For example, we can see a square table as a circular table that has sharpened its curves into corners, or a circular table as a square table that has curved its angles into arcs. Or we can see a table as having exactly the same center point, whether it's square or circular. Both tables have something in common, so they're not mutually exclusive.

In other words, any one entity, including a human being, is given its dynamic nature not by having a particular quality *instead* of its opposite, but by having a particular balance of opposite qualities. For example, among human attributes, physical strength and masculinity are considered Yang qualities, while emotional force and femininity are considered Yin qualities. Nevertheless, men are also emotional (Yin within Yang) and women are also physically strong (Yang within Yin). Indeed, no man is exclusively masculine, and no woman is exclusively feminine. Carl Jung popularized this notion in the West by referring to the "inner woman" in every man's psyche as the "anima," and the "inner man" in every woman's psyche as the "animus." Psychological well-being for men and women is a balance of the anima and the animus.

Because there is no absolute Yin or Yang in nature, everything lies along a circular continuum of opposites. Let's use the night/day pair of opposites to illustrate this point. Think of it this way: midnight, the deepest point of the night, is also the start of the next day; while noon, the highest point of the day, is also the beginning of the night.

22

Western medicine actually supports the notion of a physical Yin-Yang cycle without acknowledging it as such. Many of our biochemical and physiological functions, for example, follow a day-night balance system. Our metabolism slows down at night (the Yin period), so that we breathe slower, our blood pressure drops, our hearts beat slower, and we use up fewer calories for sleeping. Meanwhile, many biochemicals, such as hormones, are produced in larger quantities to equip us for activities during the day (the Yang period), when the other functions pick up speed.

In Chinese medicine, maintaining good human health is a matter of properly balancing the opposites—the Yin and the Yang—in every aspect of one's physical, emotional, and behavioral being. It means, for example, balancing activity during the day with rest at night. It also means helping the Yin and the Yang processes or systems in the body to operate in a harmonious way.

Physiologically, Qi is Yang (a kind of fiery energy similar in Western terms to the metabolic "burning" of calories), while blood and other body fluids are Yin. Yang organs include the "hollow" ones, such as the Small Intestine, Bladder, Large Intestine, Stomach, and Gallbladder. Yin organs are the "denser" ones, like the Heart, Kidney, Lung, Spleen/Pancreas, and Liver.

Illness can be caused by a Yin-Yang imbalance that is often characterized either as a deficiency condition (e.g., not enough Yin) or an excess condition (e.g., too much Yin). Many of the Chinese treatments that this book recommends for specific illnesses are aimed at restoring a particular kind of Yin-Yang balance, such as strengthening (or, to use the Chinese medical term, "tonifying") certain Yin factors to help alleviate a certain excess Yang condition.

Western medicine has an analogous approach to describing and treating illnesses but uses a scientific frame of reference. In Western terms, a deficiency or excess condition is referred to as the hypofunctioning or hyperfunctioning of a certain organ system. For example, a hypofunctioning adrenal gland would have signs compatible with a Yang deficiency condition, while a hyperfunctioning thyroid gland would indicate a Yang excess condition.

The Five Elements: Our Link to the Universe

Western and Chinese medicines have very different models for describing how the body works. Neither explains it all, but one thing is certain: knowing only one of them gives us a much more limited understanding of human health than knowing both of them, and having more understanding translates into better health care.

According to Western medicine, the human body follows biologic patterns of cell division and the formation of organs and tissues. Every noncellular substance in the body—such as sodium, calcium, or glucose—has a precise biochemical molecular structure. All physiological processes are described as a series of biochemical reactions, and the health of the body as a whole can be measured scientifically in terms of homeostasis: all cells and organs operating efficiently as programmed. This functioning scenario is essentially independent of all other beings and of Nature.

Chinese medicine takes a different perspective. It assumes a much more intimate relationship between human beings and the rest of the natural world (including other human beings). The Five Elements that they all have in common are Water, Wood, Fire, Earth, and Metal. In any individual's physical and emotional makeup, the Five Elements must collectively be well balanced as well as be in harmony with the rest of the natural world to ensure optimum health.

The Five Elements correspond to different parts of the body and mind. They also function symbolically to represent different aspects of a person's being. In chapter 2 we'll look at how the

Five Elements relate to different systems in our body, thereby influencing our mental, emotional, and even spiritual health.

The Mind-Body-Spirit Connection

Western medicine is primarily a physical medicine, regarding and treating human beings as fundamentally physical beings. Herein lies its strength as well as its weaknesses. For all its success in identifying, explaining, and manipulating physical situations, it tends to leave out mental, emotional, and spiritual ones. When a physical cause cannot be established for a symptom, it is declared "psychosomatic," which, in many instances, gets unfairly translated into "nonexistent."

In Chinese medicine, the human being is an integral composition of body, mind, and spirit. They can't be considered separately from each other, as they have been for centuries not only in Western medicine, but also in Western culture, philosophy, and religion. Nor can they be given blanket priorities in the treatment of illness, as they tend to receive in the West. As an example, Chinese doctors believe that emotional issues (part of Mind) can be even more important than physical ones in many chronic illnesses.

Actually, the Chinese don't categorize the various dimensions of human existence in precisely the same way that Westerners do. The Mind and the Body consist of three treasures of Life: Mind, Qi, and Essence. They correspond symbolically to the triad of Heaven, Man, and Earth; hence a familiar expression in Chinese culture, "Man is a being between Heaven and Earth."

Qi, as we've already discussed, involves physical organs and structures, such as the Western concept of the body, but it's also a metaphysical life force. One aspect of this might be called "spirit" by Westerners, in the sense of an energetic force, but that isn't quite what the term Spirit means in Chinese medicine, as we shall see. Mind, which resides in the Heart system, refers not only to intelligence, memory, and emotions (which are given far more importance than they are in Western medicine), but also to Spirit.

From a Chinese perspective, Spirit does not have religious connotations. It refers to the two souls that all of us have as part of our being: the Corporeal Soul (the soul of our body) and the Ethereal Soul (the eternal, collective soul). The Corporeal Soul comes to us at birth and dies with us. The Ethereal Soul connects us with the eternal, collective soul world, the one that all human beings have in common (and that, we tap e.g., in dreams). These two souls are associated with certain organ systems in the body: the Ethereal Soul with the Liver system, and the Corporeal Soul with the Lung system. We'll examine this connection—and the nature of these two souls—more closely in chapter 2.

Essence, a Yin substance, resides in the Kidney and affects our development, our sexual functions, and our aging process. Essence contains what we've received from our ancestors, which correlates to the Western concept of genetic inheritance.

Hands-on Health Care

In Western medicine, the primary treatments involve chemical medications and/or surgery. As effective as this approach often can be, it requires heavy reliance on outside professionals, which frequently can leave patients and caregivers feeling helpless and hopeless to contribute to their own well-being. Chinese medicine, based on the four interrelated concepts I've just outlined, equips any person to take personal and family health care responsibility more fully into his or her own hands.

I've already touched on the importance that Chinese medicine attaches to dietary management in treating illnesses. It believes that every kind of food has medicinal value, according to how it relates to the Five Elements noted earlier. I'll explain this aspect of food more specifically in chapter 3. For now let me assure you that the treatments for particular illnesses described in this book involve simple, widely available foods, easy food preparation, and flexible menu-planning.

Another hands-on aspect of Chinese medicine is that it helps us maintain health or treat illness by making small, practical, and yet very constructive adjustments in day-to-day life. As you'll discover in this book, many of the suggested changes are as easy and, ultimately, as pleasurable as periodically taking a few deep breaths, engaging in some simple physical motions, or relaxing in various especially beneficial ways.

One of Chinese medicine's most effective hands-on techniques, however, depends literally on our hands: acupressure. Manually pressing key points on the body is a form of healing that dates back at least five thousand years. Many specific points were revealed over centuries of human experience as the spots that became tender during the course of an illness or that alleviated symptoms when they were massaged.

For example, ancient foot soldiers gradually realized that a certain spot on their leg was always particularly tender after hours of marching. They found that massaging the spot often gave them a surge of energy—enough to march a few more miles. As a result, it is currently known in Chinese medicine as the "Leg Three Mile" point. It not only relieves local pain in the legs but also helps with digestive problems and strengthens the immune system (which has earned it the modern title "Master of Immunity").

Scientific studies have now demonstrated that Qi flow possesses electromagnetic properties and that acupressure/acupuncture points are small areas close to the surface of the body that conduct electricity more readily than others. Stimulating these points can result in a change in electromagnetic energy and, therefore, in Qi flow. When you massage a point in a clockwise direction, energy goes into it. When you massage in a counter-clockwise direction, energy comes out. As you'll learn in this book, illnesses characterized as "deficient" require the former kind of massage, while illnesses characterized as "excess" require the latter. At the beginning of chapter 6 you'll find easy guidelines for performing acupressure on yourself or another person, and later, each illness-related entry tells you exactly what specific points to massage.

Chinese medicine complements Western medicine. Chinese medicine not only provides a wider range of perspectives on human health but also gives us a much larger personal role in tending it. No matter what lifestyle we lead, what environment we live in, or what illness we're treating, we can develop a better, more beneficial understanding of our own natural selves and the natural selves of the people we love through Chinese medicine. As we do, we can also learn to care for ourselves and others more effectively. It's an exciting, highly gratifying endeavor, and the power to do it lies right in your hands!

CHAPTER 2

The East-West Organ Systems

Both Chinese medicine and Western medicine describe the human body in terms of organ systems. While the two classifications have much in common, including the names of the major organs, they also have significant differences. It's helpful to look briefly at *both* models, not only to gain more information about health problems but also to appreciate more fully why combining the East-West treatments recommended in this book can be so effective.

In Western medicine, organs and other physical structures are grouped into a system according to their structural and physiologic similarities. Although different systems are interrelated through blood flow and nerve supplies, they are regarded as separate entities that can be treated by medical specialists independently from other organ systems. Specific emotions are not associated with any particular system, except in terms of the psychosomatic symptoms they produce: one depressed patient may have stomach symptoms, while another may complain of headaches. The classification of organ systems and the corresponding medical specialists who treat them appear on page 31.

Let's use a patient named Jason as an example. Jason sees a pulmonologist for his lingering cough. He has some stomach symptoms that seem to get worse when he eats on the run, skips meals, and eats too much junk food, so he is thinking about seeing a gastroenterologist as well. He tells the pulmonologist that his cough gets worse when he's under unusual stress at work and that lately he has become depressed easily. The doctor does the appropriate lab tests and gives him a prescription medication for his cough. In addition, the doctor tells him that his stomach symptoms are psychosomatic and sends him to a psychiatrist, who also can treat him for his mild depression.

Jason would get a different perspective on his health problems from Chinese medicine, as we shall see later. (Chinese medicine uses the same names as Western medicine for primary organs, such as Lung, Heart, Kidney. In this book, Chinese organs are capitalized to differentiate from Western organs.)

While the organ systems are separate, independent entities in Western medicine, the twelve Chinese organ systems are intimately related to one another in two ways: (1) as Yin-Yang organ couplets that correspond to the same Element; and (2) as organs that have both nurturing and destructive associations with other organs in the Five-Element cycle. Let's look at these relationships.

Yin-Yang Organ Couplets

Each of the six Yin-Yang organ couplets consists of one Yin organ and one Yang organ. The Yin organs are the Spleen/Pancreas, Heart, Lung, Kidney, Pericardium/Master of the Heart, and Liver. They're dense in nature and carry out the physiological

Organ System and Medical Specialist

Organ Systems	Primary Organ	Other Structures	Specialists
cardiovascular	heart	pericardium, blood vessels	cardiologist
respiratory	lung	nose, airways	pulmonologist
digestive/ gastrointestinal	stomach	mouth, esophagus, liver, small intestine, large intestine	gastroenterologist
nervous system	brain	spinal cord, nerves, autonomic nervous system	neurologist
endocrine system	thyroid	hormone-secreting glands: pituitary, adrenal, gonads	endocrinologist
urinary system	kidney	bladder, collecting ureters, male genitals	nephrologist, urologist
hematopoietic system	spleen	blood cells, platelets, lymphs	hematologist
skin	skin	hair, nails, sweat glands	dermatologist
eyes	eyes	eyelids, nerves, tear ducts	ophthalmologist
ear, nose, throat	ear, nose, throat		ENT otolaryngologist
		women: pregnancy, female organs	obstetrician/ gynecologist
		mental-emotional	psychiatrist
skeletal system	bones, joints		orthopedist
all structures	all		oncologist

processes of producing, transforming, directing, and moving Qi. The Yang organs are the Stomach, Small Intestine, Large Intestine, Bladder, Triple Heater (a division of the body into three cavities without a distinct anatomical organ), and Gallbladder. They're hollow in nature and primarily carry out the functions of storage and transport. In terms of body function, they're considered less important than the Yin organs. The Yin-Yang organs are coupled as follows: Lung-Large Intestine, Spleen/Pancreas-Stomach, Heart-Small Intestine, Kidney-Bladder, Pericardium (Master of the Heart)-Triple Heater, and Liver-Gallbladder. The channels of the Yin-Yang organs connect with each other, so that the first point on the Large Intestine channel follows the last point on the Lung channel, and the last point on the Stomach channel connects to the first point on the Spleen channel, and so on. Both the Yin and Yang organs in a couplet belong to the same Element and therefore share the same human and natural correspondences. The organ systems are also related according to Five-Element interactions, which I discuss in more detail below and throughout the book. The table on page 33 summarizes the Elements, their Yin-Yang organs, and the human and natural correspondences.

The Organs and the Five Elements

Now let's look at how the Five Elements relate to one another in the natural world and in our being. Each element is the nurturer of another element and yet at the same time is the controller/destroyer of another element. We'll examine the nurturing cycle first. It operates as each element nurtures the succeeding element. The nurturer is the Mother element to the nurtured, Son element:

- Water feeds Wood, as all trees need water to grow.
- Wood provides the substance for Fire.

The Five Elements, Their Yin-Yang Organs, and Other Correspondences

Correspondences	Water	Wood	Fire	Earth	Metal
HUMAN CORRESPONDENCES					
Yin	Kidney	Liver	Heart, Pericardium	Spleen/ Pancreas	Lung
Yang	Bladder	Gall-bladder	Small Intestine, Triple Heater	Stomach	Large Intestine
emotion	will, fear	anxiety, irritability	joy, passion	introspection, sympathy	sadness
exaggerated emotions	paranoia	smoldering anger	mania, explosive anger	excess worry, obsession	depression
voice	moaning, groaning	shouting	laughing	singing	weepy sobbing
color preference	dark blue, black	Liver: blue GB: green	red	yellow Earth tones	white
taste	salty	sour	bitter	sweet	spicy
opens to orifice	ears	eyes	tongue	mouth	nose
NATURE CORRESPONDENCES					
season	winter	spring	summer	late-summer harvest	autumn
time of day	night	sunrise	noon	afternoon	sunset
direction	north	east	south	center	west
external vulnerabilities	cold	wind	heat	dampness	dryness

Five-Element Diagram

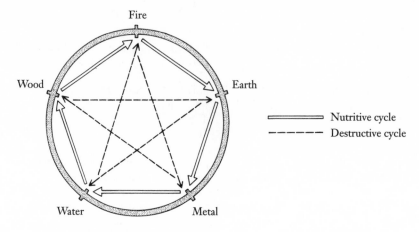

- Fire creates the ashes that become Earth.
- Earth stores Metal.
- Metal can be transformed into Water. (This is true for metals being melted down to liquid and, from a Western medical perspective, for biochemical processes such as the metabolism of glucose, or sugar, which gives off water as an end product.)

Within the human body, the Mother organs nurture the Son organs to make sure they do not become too weak or too deficient:

- Kidney (Water) nurtures Liver (Wood).
- Liver (Wood) nurtures Heart (Fire).
- Heart (Fire) nurtures Spleen/Pancreas (Earth).
- Spleen/Pancreas (Earth) nurtures Lung (Metal).
- Lung (Metal) nurtures Kidney (Water).

Each element also has a controlling or a destructive relationship with another element, which gives Five-Element interactions a sort of check-and-balance system to make sure that no one element becomes too excessive or too strong:

- Water puts out Fire.
- Fire melts Metal.
- Metal destroys Wood, as when an ax cuts down a tree.
- Wood breaks up Earth, as when a root tears into the ground
- Earth controls Water, comparable to the land defining the shapes of oceans and lakes.

Within the human body, the controlling organ prevents the controlled one from becoming excessed and, as a result, throwing the body into a state of imbalance:

- Kidney (Water) controls Heart (Fire).
- Heart (Fire) controls Lung (Metal).
- Lung (Metal) controls Liver (Wood).
- Liver (Wood) controls Spleen/Pancreas (Earth).
- Spleen/Pancreas (Earth) controls Kidney (Water).

Now you can understand why Chinese medicine takes into account a person's whole being rather than certain specialized parts. Remember Jason, the patient we looked at earlier in terms of Western medicine? Although Jason's cough is primarily a symptom of the Lungs, it can also be due to an imbalance involving the digestive system or Spleen/Pancreas (Earth) and Liver (Wood). Lung functioning can become deficient from lack of nurturance if the Spleen/Pancreas is weakened because Jason doesn't eat properly. The result can be a cough. In addition, stress can make the Liver become excessed. When the Liver goes into this state, the Lung has to work extra hard to control it and becomes weaker in the process. Jason's cough, therefore, gets even worse with stress. As his Lung weakens, sadness (the emotion associated with Metal/Lung) increases. A Chinese physician would devise a treatment plan to balance Jason's Lung, Spleen/Pancreas, and Liver. The doctor may even include treatments for other organs that may eventually be affected through the Five-Element interactions.

Now let's look at each organ in greater detail. This will

provide you with good background information for the treatment suggestions in chapter 6. We'll start with the more important Yin organs: the Lung, Kidney, Liver, Heart, and Spleen/Pancreas. Then we'll examine the less important Yang organs that correspond, respectively, with the Yin organs: the Large Intestine, Bladder, Gallbladder, Small Intestine, and Stomach. For each organ, we'll consider the physiological characteristics and functions, the emotional associations, and the Five-Element correspondences.

Yin Organs

Lung

In Western medicine, the lungs belong to the respiratory system, which is responsible for the exchange of air in the body. Air comes in through the nostrils or the mouth, moves down the windpipe (the trachea), to the air tubes in the chest (the bronchi and bronchioles), and finally to the lung tissue. When we breathe in, we take in oxygen. When we breathe out, we get rid of carbon dioxide.

In Chinese medicine, the Lung takes in pure Qi from the air and gets rid of impure Qi from our body. The Lung and Spleen/Pancreas (digestive system) have a close relationship: the pure Qi from the air combines with the Qi from food to form the nourishing Qi that circulates in our bodies. After forming Qi, the Lung then has the important function of governing or overseeing its movement through the body. The external orifice for the Lung is the nose. This entire concept correlates to the Western concept of the intake of air through the nose, the circulation of oxygen through the body, and the incorporation of oxygen into all physiologic metabolism.

In Western medicine, the lungs and the kidneys have a close relationship in maintaining the proper acid-base balance for physiologic activities in the cells and tissues. Just as the body needs to maintain a certain temperature for health, so the cells need to have just the right amount of acid and base substances to function. The lungs contribute to this balance through breathing out carbon dioxide. An imbalance can result in adverse conditions called respiratory acidosis or alkalosis. The kidneys help preserve the balance by excreting hydrogen ions. An imbalance here can result in metabolic acidosis or alkalosis.

An intimate relationship between the Lung and the Kidney also exists in Chinese medicine, in terms of the proper movement of Qi. Just as blood needs to flow in a certain direction, so does Qi in order for the systems of the body to be healthy. The Lung moves Qi in the downward direction, and the Kidney keeps it from moving upward abnormally. Wheezing and vomiting occur when Qi strays upward. In biochemical terms, wheezing can result in a respiratory acid-base imbalance, and vomiting can result in a metabolic acid-base imbalance.

While recognizing that the skin also "breathes," Western medicine considers the skin to be a separate organ from the lungs. Chinese medicine incorporates the Skin as the external aspect of the Lung. The close relationship between the Lung and the Skin is evidenced by the frequent occurrence of both respiratory and skin symptoms during the same illness. We see the identical pattern among some Western-designated illnesses; for example, eczema often accompanies asthma.

In Western medicine, the skin functions as a protective and regulating organ. It acts as a protective barrier against the physical environment, chemicals, and infection. The sweat glands within it regulate body temperature: when the internal temperature is high, the skin pores open to allow sweat to come to the surface; the evaporation of sweat cools down the body. In Chinese medicine, the Lung controls the movement of all Qi, including Defensive Qi that circulates under the skin and acts as a protective shield against "external evils." The Lung Qi also directs fluid movement to the muscles and skin and therefore controls sweating.

Lung corresponds with the element Metal. Metal symbolically represents organization and manifests in the body as the rhythmic regularity of breathing and the specific molecular structure of molecules. The emotions associated with Metal are sadness and grief. When our Lung is in a healthy state of balance, we are organized and feel normal sadness if it's appropriate for a situation. When our Lung is not in balance, we have trouble getting organized and tend to feel sad and maybe even depressed. The taste corresponding with Metal/Lung is pungent or spicy, like the taste of fumes given off by burning metal.

The Lung is also of paramount importance in housing the Corporeal Soul, the Soul of our physical body that enters us at birth and dies with us. It is closely linked in Chinese medicine to an entity called Essence, which resides in the Kidneys and, among other things, transmits qualities and information from our ancestors. The Corporeal Soul gives us our physical sensations, both in health and in illness, which explains how the itchiness of eczema can be associated with Lung disorders. Our other Soul, the Ethereal Soul, resides in the Liver Yin. It also enters our body at birth, forms our connection with other Souls during our lifetime, and returns to the Soul World after our death. These two Souls define our Spirit, making us whole beings of Body, Mind, *and* Spirit. They have no religious connotation and therefore no parallel in Western thought.

In Western medicine, the most common disorders that affect the lungs are infections. Upper respiratory tract infections (URI) are located in the nose and throat. Lower respiratory tract infections are named according to location: laryngitis, tracheitis, bronchitis, bronchiolitis, and pneumonia (infection in lung tissue). The majority of the infections are due to viruses and bacteria. The respiratory system is also vulnerable to allergens, resulting in symptoms such as congestion and sneezing in the upper tract and asthmatic wheezing in the lower tract. Chronic, severe asthma and cigarette smoking may result in emphysema, the trapping of air in the chest. Cigarettes also are the major cause of lung cancer, which is the leading cause of cancer deaths.

In Chinese medicine, Lung is vulnerable to cold and dryness. Lung symptoms are due to deficient or excess Lung Qi, to the reversal of the proper downward movement of Qi, and/or to the Lung's relationship with other energy channels. Emotionally, the symptoms may include sadness or depression. When the Corporeal Soul is disturbed, we may have a vague, general feeling of physical uneasiness, as if we are "crawling under our own skin."

Kidney

In Western medicine the kidneys have many responsibilities. They form and excrete urine. They secrete the hormones that regulate blood pressure and stimulate the production of red blood cells. The kidneys and lungs share the important responsibility of maintaining acid-base balance. In the above discussion of the lungs, I mentioned that the cells in our body need to have just the right amount of acid and base substances to function. The kidneys help in this process by controlling the excretion of salt and hydrogen ions. Insufficient kidney function results in disorders called metabolic acidosis or alkalosis.

In Chinese medicine, the Kidney performs some of the same characteristic functions but also others that have no parallel in Western medicine. The Kidney is the foundation of life. Although it is a Yin organ, it is the root of Qi and of Yin and Yang for all the organs. The Kidney also stores Essence *(Jing)*, a substance without a Western equivalent.

Jing exerts powerful effects for the entire body that include growth, development, maturation, sexual function, conception, pregnancy, childbirth, and aging. Jing also transmits qualities and information from one generation to the next (what Western medicine calls genetic inheritance). Jing is precious and not easily replaced. So-called pre-Heaven Jing is inherited. Post-Heaven Jing can come from food and can be augmented by special Qi exercises, such as Qigong or Tai Chi.

Jing is quickly expended with stress, with aging, and with ejaculation in the male and menstruation in the female. The state of our head hair reflects the state of our Kidney Qi, which explains not only the gradual graying of hair as we age and depletion of our Jing, but also the sudden or accelerated graying in individuals who experience severe physical or emotional shock.

The Kidney opens to the ear. Western medicine regards the ear and the kidneys as separate organs and cannot explain the many health-related associations between the two. For example, people with congenital kidney anomalies often have low-set ears; and some antibiotics, such as Gentamycin, can be toxic to both the ears and the kidneys. Chinese medicine easily explains these situations as relating, respectively, to deficient Kidney Jing and to Kidney Qi injury.

The Kidney includes marrow in its realm of influence. However, the interpretation of marrow between the two disciplines is worlds apart. The marrow in Western medicine is responsible for the production of antibodies, red and white blood cells, and platelets. The marrow in Chinese medicine includes the spinal cord and the brain, called the "sea of marrow." Therefore, in Western medicine the brain, which distinguishes man as a superior, intellectual being, is just a "curious organ" in Chinese medicine that depends on Kidney Qi.

As in Western medicine, the Kidney in Chinese medicine has a close relationship with the Lung. However, the Chinese explain this relationship in terms of the movement of Qi: the Lung controls the movement of Qi downward, and the Kidney grasps the Qi and prevents abnormal flow upward. When Kidney Qi is deficient, the downward flow of Lung Qi is disrupted. Qi then moves upward and manifests as wheezing or vomiting.

The Kidney is associated with the Water Element. In both

Western and Chinese medicine, the Kidney is responsible for fluid and water balance in the body. The taste corresponding with Water/Kidney Qi is salt, which has a profound effect on fluid volume in the body. The emotion associated with the Kidney is willpower when Kidney Qi is balanced and fear when Kidney Qi is out of balance. A healthy dose of fear can keep us from taking foolish risks. When Kidney Qi is unbalanced, we may appear to lack the willpower to be decisive but in reality we are scared. There is an ebb-and-flow, waterlike quality to this indecisiveness. For example, someone with Kidney Qi deficiency may have trouble making a commitment to marry. Fear from Kidney deficiency may become so great that it prevents normal emotional growth or escalates concern about insignificant things. For example, most of us have known an elderly person who has exaggerated fears and insecurities about small, even inconsequential matters. This can happen to all of us, as our Kidney Qi and Essence diminish with age.

In Western medicine, kidney problems are due to the inadequate formation or excretion of urine, and to toxicity from the accumulation of waste products. Disorders of the kidney include infections-(e.g., glomerulonephritis, pyelonephritis); nephrosis; kidney stones; kidney involvement in the immune disorder systemic lupus; and cancer. Treatments include medication and dialysis. According to Western medicine, most people can function with one kidney. Therefore, unlike other transplants, kidney transplants can come from live donors.

In Chinese medicine, Kidney never has excess disorders, since we can always use more Kidney Qi and Jing. The deficiency disorders can be in Kidney Yin or Kidney Yang or both. Since the Kidney is the root of all organs, it is often affected by imbalances in other organs, resulting in multiple organ deficiencies, such as Kidney-Lung deficiency and Kidney-Liver deficiency. Treatment always involves tonification or strengthening (never sedation) of the Kidney and other involved organs.

Liver

The liver is the largest internal organ in the body. The liver gets oxygenated blood from the heart, and nutrients from the digestive system. The liver is a very versatile organ and has a long list of metabolic and secretory functions. Chinese medicine agrees about its overall importance to body functioning and calls Liver the "General" of the Qi system. It is Liver that directs smooth and proper Qi movement in all directions.

Biochemically, the list of liver functions includes the breakdown of bilirubin, the secretion of bile, and the metabolism of carbohydrates, fat, drugs, and hormones. The liver is also involved in the immune function and detoxification of the body. The liver stores glycogen, vitamins, iron, and minerals; and it produces protein and clotting factors. The liver also synthesizes cholesterol. Many of these processes generate heat for maintaining our body temperature.

This precise biochemical description of the liver is complemented by the Chinese metaphoric and symbolic description of Liver. Liver is a Wood organ. Think of it as a young tree, as springtime with everything in bloom. All the metabolic processes in the body are aimed toward growth and maturation, just like a sapling evolving into a full-fledged tree. Liver Qi is responsible for lubricating tendons, ligaments, and muscles. When Liver Qi is well balanced, we feel youthful, we can move about freely and gracefully, we blossom. When our Liver Qi is unhealthy, we feel stiff, like a piece of old wood.

Western medicine tells us that the liver contains about 10 percent of the blood in the body and carries blood from the pancreas and the spleen. In Chinese medicine the Liver stores blood, regulates the quantity of blood and fluid, and, in women, regulates menstruation.

Western medicine does not relate any sort of emotional functioning to the liver. Chinese medicine associates Liver with frustration, irritability, and anxiety—the emotions of an impatient child. When Liver Qi is out of balance, these emotions become exaggerated. A person suffering from such a condition can experience smoldering anger accompanied by resentment and even withdrawal. As the General, Liver Qi enables us to have a good sense of direction in our lives, just as a healthy tree grows straight and tall. When Liver Qi is unbalanced, we don't know which direction to take. We feel angry, confused, and lost. Resenting everything, we may withdraw and become quiet or even depressed.

The Liver has another very important role according to Chinese medicine: Liver Yin houses our Ethereal Soul. This Soul loosely correlates to the Western concept of a soul as an eternal being, but Soul from a Chinese perspective has no religious connotation. Like its physical counterpart the Corporeal Soul, which resides in the Lung, the Ethereal Soul enters our body at birth. Unlike the Corporeal Soul, this Ethereal Soul "visits" the Soul world when we dream and leaves our body when we die to return to the Soul world and enters another physical being. This Soul influences our thinking and our emotions, which in Chinese medicine is called Mind. Therefore it is closely related to the Heart, which houses Shen, the Chinese term that translates as both Spirit and Mind. Through the Ethereal Soul, our Mind becomes connected with other minds, and we can access thoughts and ideas from eternity. In this way it is more closely related to the Jungian concept of our collective unconscious, which is made up of the individual unconscious from each of us.

The external orifices associated with Liver are the eyes. This explains why liver symptoms often appear first in the eyes, such as the eyes turning yellow before the skin does in a case of jaundice. The taste associated with Wood/Liver is sour—the taste of bile.

From a Western perspective, the most common disorder of the liver is hepatitis (inflammation of the liver), which usually is caused by viral infection, but may also be triggered by bacteria, parasites, chemical agents, or drugs. Although most cases of hepatitis are self-limiting, a small percentage may lead to chronic hepatitis and cirrhosis (scarring of the liver). Chronic alcoholism can lead to alcoholic cirrhosis. Jaundice comes from built-up deposits of bilirubin when the diseased liver cannot break it down. Excess fat can lead to fatty degeneration of the liver. Liver cancer usually is caused by cancer spreading from some other area. In a small percentage of cases, liver conditions are due to congenital anomalies. The treatment of liver problems varies greatly, depending on the nature of the disorder. Over the past two decades, liver transplants have been successful even in children.

From a Chinese perspective, Liver Qi usually becomes stagnant but never deficient. The Chinese Liver is highly susceptible to Wind, just as a small tree sways back and forth in the wind. What the Chinese call "internal wind" characterizes many disorders that "do not stay in one place," such as seizures. Liver Qi stagnation is associated with pain, such as headaches or pain below the rib cage. Liver Blood and Liver Yin can become deficient, resulting in symptoms such as dizziness, muscle spasms, and weakness. The emotions mentioned above may manifest in varying degrees with all of the disorders. When the Ethereal Soul is also affected, we may appear to be not "with it." We cannot think clearly, cannot perform our jobs, and just in general do not seem to be able to get going.

Spleen/Pancreas

In Western medicine, the spleen and the pancreas are considered to be distinctly different organs, although they are in close anatomical contact. The spleen is primarily a blood organ involved in removing iron from the hemoglobin of red blood cells (RBC) and clearing old red blood cells from the bloodstream. The spleen also stores RBCs and releases them in times of need, such as when the body is bleeding. In addition, the spleen manufactures antibodies and helps remove waste products. The pancreas secretes insulin to regulate blood sugar. Diabetes results from an elevation of blood sugar (hyperglycemia) due to an insulin deficiency.

In Chinese medicine, Spleen and Pancreas are incorporated into one entity, which will be called Spleen/Pancreas throughout this book. The Spleen/Pancreas carries out similar functions involving digestion and blood. The Spleen/Pancreas is the Yin organ of the digestive couplet, the Stomach being the Yang organ. Food "rots and ripens" in the Stomach, which correlates to the Western concept of food being broken down by stomach acid and enzymes. The Spleen/Pancreas has the important function of transforming food into Qi and then transporting Qi, nutrients, and fluid to the other organs. It also nourishes the muscles and the limbs with Qi. When our Spleen/Pancreas Qi is strong, we have a lot of physical energy. When it is weak, we feel tired.

The Spleen/Pancreas "governs" blood and is therefore responsible for "holding" blood in blood vessels. In a case of Spleen/Pancreas deficiency, there may be menstrual difficulties and abnormal bleeding. The Spleen/Pancreas Qi also has a "lifting" effect of the organs to make sure they stay in place; otherwise the organs can prolapse. A prolapse of the rectum, for example, causes a hemorrhoid.

Spleen/Pancreas corresponds to the Earth Element. It makes sense that the digestive system is symbolically associated with Mother Earth, the provider of nourishment to all living beings. It also corresponds in Nature with late summer, which is the harvest season. Earth's taste is sweet, the predominant flavor in fruits and vegetables. This means that eating normal amounts of naturally sweetened food is healthy, while consuming an excessive amount of sweet foods—especially artificially sweetened foods—can throw the digestive system out of balance.

The mental functions associated with Spleen/Pancreas are

thinking and introspection. The emotional function is sympathy, a characteristic commonly attributed to mothers. When we have well-balanced Earth/Digestive Qi, we feel centered, we can think clearly, and we can be sympathetic. When our Earth/ Digestive Qi is unbalanced, we cannot think clearly, we worry a lot, and we can even become obsessive and self-absorbed in extreme circumstances.

The Spleen/Pancreas is susceptible to dampness, so treatment guidelines often involve controlling or alleviating dampness. The external orifice for this system is the mouth—tasting, chewing, and preparing food for further digestion.

In Western medicine, the spleen is frequently involved in all sorts of infections: viral, bacterial, parasitic, and others. It is easily traumatized and has to be surgically removed when it hemorrhages. The spleen seldom has cancerous growths. The pancreas, however, can develop cancer more easily, although it is not as susceptible to infections and trauma.

In Chinese medicine, Spleen/Pancreas problems usually manifest as deficiencies. Dampness, poor diet, and overwork are the triggers. The symptoms can range from fatigue, paleness, and muscle weakness to various digestive-related difficulties such as loss of appetite, a bloating sensation in the abdomen, or diarrhea. The Spleen/Pancreas also can be involved secondarily with disorders of the Lung and Liver, the two organs related to it in the nutritive and destructive cycles. Treatment of any Spleen/Pancreas illness usually consists of tonification or strengthening.

Heart

From a Western perspective, the heart is a mechanical pump that is closely associated with the lungs. The heart pumps blood to the lungs for oxygenation, then pumps oxygenated blood throughout the body. When the heart stops, death ensues. In rare circumstances the heart can be replaced with a transplant.

Chinese medicine regards the Heart as the "Emperor," the irreplaceable organ that rules the body in all aspects of our being: physical, emotional, and spiritual. On a physical level, the Heart governs the movement of blood in the blood vessels and is closely related to the Lung in that Qi and blood nourish each other. It is the vitality of Qi within the blood vessels that moves blood. Our facial complexion reflects the condition of our Heart: Rosy cheeks indicate good blood flow and a healthy Heart, while a pale complexion indicates anemia, poor blood flow, and an unhealthy Heart. Through the interaction of fluids and Blood, the Heart also influences sweat and other body fluids.

The Heart opens onto the tongue and therefore influences speech. When our Heart is calm, we are articulate. When our Heart is bothered, we have a hard time finding the right words. We stutter. We forget what we want to say.

The most important function of the Heart, however, is being the House for Shen. There is no precise English translation for Shen. It can mean both the Mind and the Spirit. This reflects the closeness of the Ethereal Soul (discussed above, in the Liver section) and the Mind. Through this Soul, our individual mind accesses thoughts and images of eternity from the Soul World. In this way the minds of all people are in some way connected with each other.

When the Heart is in a state of balance, the Shen is said to be properly housed. The Emperor rules wisely. We can think clearly and creatively. We have articulate speech, can experience joy and passion, and we are at peace with ourselves. We also can connect more vitally with one another. When the Heart is in a state of imbalance, the Shen is not properly housed. The Emperor is not ruling well. We are restless and distracted. We cannot think clearly and become irrational and inarticulate. We cannot remember things or sleep well. We also feel disconnected with others. In severe cases we can become hysterical and delirious or even completely lose consciousness. In a concrete sense, this state correlates physically to the Western concept of a coma caused by decreased blood flow to the brain, which occurs in instances of blocked arteries. On a mental-emotional level, it correlates to Western diagnosis of psychosis. The Heart is very vulnerable and can easily become imbalanced in any emotionally troubled situation.

The Heart's Element is Fire. The primary emotion of the Heart is joy or passion. When the Heart is in balance, we can experience normal fiery passion, as in love. When the Heart is out of balance, we can become explosive. Because all other emotions—sadness, anger, fear, worry—can eventually affect the Heart, it is the center of our emotional being. We can find the same concept expressed metaphorically in the English language; for example, "I can't do this—my heart is just not in it."

The color corresponding to the Heart is red—the color of blood, passion, and fire. The taste associated with the Heart is bitterness. When the Heart is hurt, the fiery passion can turn into bitterness.

In Western medicine, heart disorders are due to anatomic or biochemical problems, such as coronary artery disease, heart or valve malformations, infections, high blood pressure, and arrhythmia (irregular heart rhythm). Treatment usually involves medication. In cases of severe coronary artery disease, bypass surgery or, less frequently, a heart transplant, may be performed.

In Chinese medicine, Heart disorders include physical and emotional problems; both can reflect (or can be due to) deficiency of Heart blood or Qi. Heart, being the center of emotions, can become secondarily deficient due to chronic emotional problems from other organ imbalances. This causes the Heart fire to be out of control, giving rise to excess mental symptoms of agitation, restlessness, and/or physical symptoms of excess heat such as palpitations, feeling warm, or needing cold drinks.

Pericardium/Master of the Heart

The pericardium in Western medicine is simply the covering of the heart. It can develop an infection (pericarditis) that doesn't involve the heart itself.

In Chinese medicine the Pericardium is also called Master of the Heart. It assumes a significant, multifaceted role in protecting the Heart. Among other tasks, it wards off external evils and pathogens. Its title, Master of the Heart refers specifically to its influence on the heart rate. It is therefore analogous to the sympathetic nervous system in Western medicine—a system that controls involuntary functions such as heart rate. There is a great deal of overlap between the Heart and Master of the Heart, as both are associated with the Fire Element. The Pericardium channel runs next to the Heart channel along the inside of the arm. While the Heart is influenced by *all* emotions, the Master of the Heart is affected primarily by emotional difficulties pertaining to our relationships.

Yang Organs

Large Intestine

From a Western perspective, the large intestine receives wastes from the small intestine, reabsorbs some fluid, and excretes the rest. The rhythmic contraction of the intestinal muscles propels wastes down the large intestine. The most common disorders associated with it are constipation and diarrhea, which may be caused by infections from viruses, bacteria, or parasites. Ulcerative colitis is a chronic condition in which the colon wall becomes inflamed and forms ulcers. The symptoms include diarrhea, bleeding, stools with mucus, and pain.

Treatment for most large-intestine disorders includes dietary management and medication. Surgical removal is indicated in severe cases when there is no response to medication or when there is a risk for developing colon cancer, the third most common cancer in the United States.

From a Chinese perspective, the Large Intestine performs the same task of excretion as its Western counterpart. However, there are two major differences. First, the Chinese Spleen/Pancreas controls the transformation and transportation of food and fluid throughout the entire digestive system, including the Large Intestine. Many of the symptoms that a Western doctor might attribute to the large intestine, such as diarrhea or abdominal pain, are usually attributed by a Chinese doctor to Spleen/Pancreas deficiency. Second, the Large Intestine is the Yang organ coupled to Lung. When Lung Qi is deficient, there is less Qi being sent to the Large Intestine, and a person may become constipated. This is often seen in elderly people, as Lung Qi naturally weakens with age. Alternatively, if the Large Intestine does not function well, food stagnates, the Lung Qi cannot descend, and a person may develop cough or shortness of breath. The Large Intestine plays no mental-emotional role in a person's health.

Bladder

Both Western and Chinese medicine consider the Bladder as the organ for the storage and excretion of urine formed by the Kidney. The symptoms and even the causes of Bladder-related problems are described similarly by the two traditions.

In Western medicine, bedwetting (nocturnal enuresis) is considered to have a strong correlation with the emotions, especially fear. Chinese medicine explains the association of bedwetting with fear quite clearly: The Bladder is linked directly to fear along with its companion, Water/Yin organ, Kidney. Fear causes an abnormal flow of Qi, called a "sinking" of Qi in the Bladder, which manifests as bedwetting.

Western medicine explains incontinence among the elderly as the loss of sphincter control and the degeneration of nerve innervation. Chinese medicine has a slightly different but compatible explanation. Kidney Qi and Essence control aging, and both decrease as we grow older. Incontinence is the Bladder's manifestation of this condition.

The Bladder has no mental/emotional function.

Gallbladder

Western medicine describes the gallbladder as a muscular sac that stores bile secreted by the liver. When bile is needed for digestion, the gallbladder releases it into the duodenum part of the intestines.

In Chinese medicine, the Gallbladder also functions as a storehouse for bile. Together with its couplet organ Liver, it also controls the movement of tendons. Liver nourishes tendons with blood, while Gallbladder nourishes them with Qi.

The Gallbladder also coordinates with the Liver to play an important role in our mental-emotional well-being. The Liver as General gives us directions, and the Gallbladder Qi enables us to make decisions and changes in our lives. When the Gallbladder works in harmony with the Liver, we can make the decisions and the changes more confidently. When the Gallbladder is unbalanced, we become timid about venturing out in life.

According to Western medicine, the major gallbladder disorder is the formation of gallstones from the salts and cholesterol in bile. They are common among diabetics, in African Americans, and in overweight women beyond age forty. Treatment consists of taking bile salts to dissolve the stones, using ultrasound to shatter the stones, or having them surgically removed. The presence of highly concentrated bile can cause the gallbladder to become inflamed, and sometimes it can become secondarily infected. The formation of any kind of tumor in the gallbladder is very rare. Chinese medicine attributes similar problems to the Gallbladder, but they are explained in terms of excesses and deficiencies.

Small Intestine

From a Western point of view, the most extensive part of digestion occurs in the small intestine, where digested food is absorbed and where water and wastes are sent down to the large intestine. The most common disorders of the small intestine are giardia (parasitic infection), ileitis (inflammation of the small intestine), and Crohn's disease (a chronic condition of inflammation of the intestinal wall producing symptoms of diarrhea, abdominal pain, weight loss, and fever).

In Chinese medicine the Small Intestine performs digestive functions, separating (in its terms) the "clean" from the "dirty." It also has an emotional role. Metaphorically, it can be said to help us "sort things out." It assists our mind in determining what we need and don't need, so we can think clearly and make decisions. The disorders of the Small Intestine are described as excesses or deficiencies. It is especially vulnerable to the temperature of food. For example, excessive exposure to cold foods can cause a Small Intestine Qi deficiency.

Triple Heater/Triple Burner

The Triple Heater or Triple Burner is a difficult system to define in terms of Western medicine. The designation doesn't really refer to an organ but rather to three closely associated divisions of the body described below.

Nevertheless, the Triple Burner is considered a Yang organ— the couplet organ of the Yin organ—Pericardium/Master of the Heart. The Triple Burner's overall function is the regulation and circulation of body fluid. With the fluid, it nourishes, moistens, warms, and cools tissues. It acts as if it is the sum total of all the Yang organs united into one entity, and in this way gives a sense of oneness to all the Yang organs in the body. The nature of the fluid being distributed varies in each division, reflecting the physiology of the corresponding organs. The three divisions are:

UPPER BURNER

location	thorax or chest area above the diaphragm
organs	Heart, Lung, and Master of the Heart
fluid form	mist or vapor—Lung fluid distributed as a fine mist or vapor to the skin, muscles, and overall fluid circulation

MIDDLE BURNER

location	abdominal cavity above the navel
organs	Spleen/Pancreas, Stomach, Gallbladder, and Liver
fluid form	foam, turbid pool—food and drink from digestion

LOWER BURNER

location	lower abdominal cavity below the navel
organs	Small and Large Intestine, Kidney, and Bladder
fluid form	"swamp" or "drainage ditch" type of fluid—the final separation of the "clean" from the "dirty"

The Triple Burner treatment points in acupressure and acupuncture are used to maintain balance in these three divisions of the body and to bring about fluid balance in a wide range of disorders. There are no disease entities specific to the Triple Burner.

Stomach

Western diagnoses relating to stomach problems include stomach flu, indigestion, gastritis, stomach ulcers, and cancer. Treatment depends on the disorder.

In Chinese medicine, the Stomach is the most important Yang organ. It "rots and ripens" food, which is comparable to the Western concept of digesting food in the stomach.

The special importance of the Stomach is reflected in the Chinese term for digestive organs: the "Root of Post-Heaven Qi." This means that the couplet organs of Stomach and Spleen/Pancreas are the beginning of all the Qi produced in the body after birth. This couplet also has the closest relationship of all the Yin-Yang couplets. The two organs together are responsible for digesting food, extracting Qi from food, and for transporting nutritive Qi throughout the body, including the muscles of our arms and legs.

As in the Western model, the Stomach sends food to the Small Intestine. From the Chinese medical standpoint, this means that Digestive Qi must move downward. When the Stomach is healthy, food and Qi move downward from the Stomach to the Small Intestine and, finally, to the Large Intestine. When the Stomach is unbalanced, the downward Qi movement is poorly directed and Qi starts to come upward. This may result in symptoms such as burping, regurgitation, nausea, vomiting, and an uncomfortable sense of fullness. The Stomach is vulnerable to dryness, because digestion in the Stomach is optimal when there is plenty of fluid. We can often feel this when we try eating food without drinking something on the side.

The Stomach plays a minor role in our mental-emotional being compared to the pervasive influence of the Spleen/Pancreas. Sometimes we can feel confused as the result of a Stomach imbalance, but that's about as far as it goes. In contrast to this, Westerners tend to think of the stomach as being strongly linked with our mental-emotional states, mainly because Western medicine frequently can't establish any physical or biochemical basis for symptoms of stomach discomfort.

Chinese medicine maintains that the Stomach can be affected by diet, our way of eating, coldness, and dryness. Stomach disorders can manifest as both deficiency and excess conditions. Stomach functioning is also easily affected by conditions of the Spleen.

CHAPTER 3

Evaluate Your Health

We all want to improve our ability to detect and assess health problems at home before they become so serious that we need to consult medical professionals. Western medicine provides us with a few basic and reliable tools we can use, such as, scales to measure our weight, blood pressure gauges, body temperature thermometers, and a vast amount of lifestyle-management literature. Chinese medicine offers us a wealth of additional ways to make better evaluations of our own health and that of our loved ones daily.

Grounded in commonsense observation and everyday language, Chinese medicine takes into account the entire individual —physically, mentally, emotionally, and spiritually—as well as everything that he or she experiences daily. From a Chinese perspective, basic health evaluation requires only the skills of practical information-gathering and decision-making—skills that anyone can easily acquire. More sophisticated evaluations can be performed by a professional if necessary. By contrast, diagnoses in Western medicine tend to focus on specific symptoms that relate to particular, scientifically defined illnesses and that require a specialist's expertise—a situation that often causes laypeople to feel incapable of figuring out any kind of health problem on their own.

The Chinese approach to health evaluation is especially effective in assessing what Westerners call psychosomatic or partly psychosomatic illnesses. Examples are fatigue, migraine headaches, asthma, pain, upset stomach, and insomnia, to name just a few. In Western medicine these illnesses often can't be shown to *originate* in the body, although they often produce physical symptoms; they are often relegated to the mysterious world of the psyche. Chinese medicine, however, can detect and meaningfully describe such conditions even when no physical symptoms yet exist. The ability it gives us to discern potential structural damage *before* it occurs makes Chinese medicine remarkably effective in preventing illness, slowing its progress, or minimizing its eventual impact.

Western medicine deemphasizes a specific person's inner nature or character, concentrating instead on the particular illness and affected body part. Although it acknowledges the existence of a personal "temperament"—one that's apparent in a newborn and later evolves into a personality—it doesn't offer a useful system for examining this factor at home, for recognizing its relationship to health, or for accommodating it in treating health problems. Instead, Western medicine tends to consider a given diagnosis as the same illness for everyone, regardless of the person who "gets" it. Along with this illness goes one medication for all, and one dosage for all, cut in half for children because they're smaller.

Chinese medicine supplies the missing tools for addressing the sick *person* rather than the person's *sickness*. Two of its most helpful frameworks for evaluating a person's overall state of being are a Yin-Yang classification system and a Five-Element classification system.

Both systems use simple words and Nature-based metaphors to describe different types of people with different predispositions regarding health. You'll find that the more you live with these systems, the more fluently they'll speak to you, and the more they'll reveal about individual health problems and how to deal with them.

Before reading any farther, complete the following two questionnaires. Your honest responses—unprejudiced by knowing anything more about the two classification systems—will reveal your Yin-Yang type and your major Five-Element type or types. You may want to record your answers on a separate sheet of paper so that other people can complete the same questionnaires without seeing previous marks. You can reuse these questionnaires yourself to classify people you know very well, such as children in your family who are too young to complete them on their own.

Questionnaire #1

Choose only *one* response in each row—the response that comes closest to describing you. Give yourself one point for each response.

	I	II	III
I am	male	comfortable both alone and in crowds	female
I am mostly	extroverted, outgoing		introverted/not outgoing
I am most energetic	during the day	both day and night	during the night
I work	a lot, like a workaholic	some balance work/play	a little
I exercise	a lot	regularly	a little
My complexion is	reddish	pink	pale
I usually feel	hot	average: not too hot or too cold	cold
I like	cold liquids	sometimes warm, sometimes cold liquids	warm/hot liquids
I am	domineering	neither domineering nor passive	passive
I am	easily angered	angry sometimes	seldom angry

My voice is	loud	average in volume	soft
My mouth/skin tend to be	dry	normal in moisture	moist
I get upset	all the time	sometimes	seldom
I get angry	all the time	sometimes	seldom
I speak my mind	all the time	sometimes	seldom
I get depressed	seldom	sometimes	a lot
I cry	seldom	sometimes	easily
I have	a very good appetite	an average appetite	a poor appetite
I am	energetic	tired when I do a lot	tired a lot
I gain weight	not easily	when I eat a lot	easily
I tend to have	constipation	normal stools	loose stools

Score _____   _____   _____

Questionnaire #2

Choose *all* items that apply to you, even if it means more than one item in the same box or more than one column in the same row. Give yourself one point for each response.

	A	B	C	D	E
My age is	under twelve years	teenage	twenties to mid-thirties	middle-aged	elderly
My favorite color is	green-blue	red	yellow	white	navy blue, black; pastel
My favorite season is	spring	summer	late summer	autumn	winter
I am vulnerable to (dislike too much of)	wind	heat	dampness	dryness	cold
My favorite flavor of food is	sour	bitter	sweet	spicy	salty
I am good at	planning things	having insight, understanding, supervising	intellectualizing, being sympathetic, calm, and generous	organizing, being methodical and meticulous	being motivated and determined
I am good at	making decisions	sorting things out	enjoying good food and company	being responsible	being level-headed

I have problems with	planning things	having insight, understanding, supervising	intellectualizing, sympathetic calm, generosity	organizing, being methodical, meticulous	being motivated, determined
I have problems with	making decisions	sorting things out	enjoying good food and company	responsibility	being level-headed
I am usually	irritable, angry, timid, shy	excitable, passionate, very happy	a frequent worrier	sad/depressed	afraid a lot, suspicious
I am also	self-conscious	talkative	introspective	honest; careful with money	analytical
At times I may be	very withdrawn	manic, explosive	obsessive	very depressed	paranoiac
My voice usually has the quality of	shouting	laughing	singing	sobbing	moaning, groaning
I tend to have	neck and shoulder pains/problems	muscle cramps, chest pain	heaviness in legs and calves	skin problems, allergies	low back pain, cold feet
I have weakness in (or am prone to infections/problems in)	eyes, eyesight	tongue, taste	mouth, lips	nose, throat	hands and ears; hearing, balance
I tend to have symptoms involving my	liver, gallbladder	heart	digestive system	lungs; immunity	kidneys, bladder
My favorite time of the day is (I am most energetic from)	11 P.M.–3 A.M.	11 A.M.–3 P.M.	7 A.M.–11 A.M.	3 A.M.–7 A.M.	3 P.M.–7 P.M.

	A	B	C	D	E
My least favorite time of the day is (I am least energetic from)	11 P.M.–3 A.M.	11 A.M.–3 P.M.	7 A.M.–11 A.M.	3 A.M.–7 A.M.	3 P.M.–7 P.M.
Compared to others of my age and sex, I am	muscular, stocky	slender	short, overweight	tall, thin	round and puffy in build
My complexion is	dark	reddish	sallow/yellowish	white	pale
My hands are	proportioned	long	short, square	long	small, puffy
My fingers are (have)	fine lines like tree markings; knotty	long, slender	short	zigzag	short
The shape of my fingernails is (resembles)	oblong	oval, pointed	triangular	rectangular	crescent-moon

Scores _____ _____ _____ _____ _____

Your Internal Yin-Yang Balance

For a moment, put aside your responses to the two questionnaires and imagine a party where the most noticeable guest is a woman named Julie, clearly the belle of the ball. Her laughter can be heard across the room, and her bright red dress stands out in a crowd of mostly dark, muted evening colors. Close up, you can see that her hands are small, but her fingers are long and slender, and her nails are oval and pointed.

Julie moves quickly among the guests, but slows down when a man catches her eye—a pale, round-faced, gray-haired man sitting alone in a corner. His navy-blue shirt and pants make him inconspicuous. "Hi, my name is Julie," she says to the man. As she shakes his hand, he can't help but compare her long fingers wrapped around his puffy hand to eagle talons wrapped around fleshy prey.

"Hi, I'm Max," he replies. His soft voice has a slight moan to it, and his glance is fleeting.

Julie senses he's somewhat uncomfortable with the encounter, and yet there's something about him that attracts her to him. She pours on the charm. After a few minutes of typical party chitchat, Max excuses himself. "I'm sorry I have to leave, I'm awfully tired and I've got to get some rest."

When Julie gives him a disappointed look, Max can't resist adding, "You know, a good, full night's rest can do wonders for insomnia and stress. You ought to try it!" As he speaks, he looks straight into her eyes and smiles, as if he knows deep, dark secrets about her life.

"How did *he* know?" she says to herself as he leaves the room. She is so shocked she forgets to be insulted. She has said nothing about her chronic inability to sleep or about all the nagging troubles that have been bothering her lately. She napped and had a facial before the party, and a glass of wine considerably brightened her mood. Several people at the party told her how well she looked and how happy she seemed. How could this quiet, retiring man possibly tell what was going on in her life?

Actually, Max could have told Julie a lot more about her simply on the basis of how she'd looked and behaved during their brief, superficial encounter. He'd surmised that she had a creative mind, a tendency toward explosive anger, a preference for warm or hot weather, and a very passionate sexual nature—all very much the opposite of him.

After you've read this book and experimented for a while with evaluating people's Yin-Yang balance, you'll be able to read people as easily as Max can. You'll even be able to read yourself and better understand yourself than you ever have before.

Modern science can analyze you by taking computerized, cross-sectional images of your body, by measuring chemicals that swim inside you, by looking at your chromosomes to tell what you've inherited and what you're capable of passing along, and by examining microscopically all the other minute structures within every single cell. Such are the marvels of modern medicine.

Ancient healers did not have these capabilities. For thousands of years, all they had were their eyes, ears, nose, tongue, hands, and mind. Through their sensory perceptions and their mental powers, they developed highly effective ways of understanding health and disease. Among the most remarkable and well-validated systems of this type is the Chinese classification of Yin or Yang characteristics in a person's physical constitution and behavior—a system that, like the Five-Elements system, has been refined over centuries of expert observations and applications.

Typical Yin characteristics, for example, include being shy, having a round or puffy body, being at rest, and feeling cold. Typical Yang characteristics are, logically, the opposite: being outgoing, having a lean or tight body, being active, and feeling hot. Once you are able to read these characteristics in an individual (including yourself), you can detect possible imbalances that may be causing—or that may eventually cause—health problems.

First let's consider Julie, and then we'll turn to the Yin-Yang questionnaire you completed. Julie is definitely extroverted, a Yang quality, plus she has other Yang attributes, such as liking the color red and having long, slender fingers, with oval, pointed nails. Putting all these details together, plus noticing her slightly hyper behavior, even for a predominantly Yang person, Max deduces that Julie probably is having excess Yang-related health problems, such as insomnia and stress.

Now let's consider questionnaire #1, which you just filled out for yourself. The three columns list Yin-Yang characteristics as follows:

- column I: Yang
- column II: balanced Yin-Yang
- column III: Yin

The highest score indicates your predominant type.

From a Chinese perspective, a major health care goal is to work toward balancing this list in your own life. For example, if your list shows that you are inclined to be very active (with many Yang characteristics such as "extroverted," "work a lot," "domineering"), then you need to take care to balance this activity with rest. As you read through this book, you'll learn other dimensions of Yin-Yang–related health care, especially in the context of treating particular kinds of illness.

The Five Elements in Human Form

Over thousands of years of observation and treatment, Chinese medical practitioners have confirmed that the basic Five Elements in the physical universe—Wood, Fire, Earth, Metal, and Water—can be used metaphorically to define five basic types of human constitutions. Each constitutional type—the Wood type, the Fire type, the Earth type, the Metal type, and the Water type—includes not only a person's physical body, but also his or her mind, spirit, behavioral predispositions, and personal preferences.

In Western terms, these types can be called "biopsychotypes." In fact, Western medicine is beginning to recognize the existence of certain biopsychotypes through tracking correspondences between a person's biochemical makeup and his or her psychological nature. Meanwhile, using the Chinese Five-Element typing system, we can assess an individual's natural tendency toward health or disease and combine that assessment with Western diagnoses to get a better, more comprehensive perspective on health care needs.

In the second questionnaire you just completed, each column lists characteristics of a different element: A = Wood, B = Fire, C = Earth, D = Metal, and E = Water. In each column, total the number of items you circled. The results tell you which element or elements predominate in your constitution.

To gain a better sense of each of the five types and some of the related health issues, let's look at sample case histories. We'll start with a Wood type named Logan.

Logan: The Wood Type

Women often cast admiring glances at Logan when he steps out of the surf at the beach or even as he walks down a city street: he is dark and muscular, with broad shoulders. At the office, his boss and colleagues usually can count on him to plan projects and make decisions. He doesn't talk much, but he works hard and gets things done. In an effort to stay fit by doing what he sees on TV, he lifts weights in the office gym, drinks orange juice all day, and usually has salad with his favorite vinaigrette dressing for both lunch and dinner.

Lately Logan is working overtime more often than not, and his behavior is taking a turn for the worse. His friends and coworkers are noticing that he gets defensive and irritable when they approach him with questions. Sometimes he broods with resentment; at other times he gets angry for no reason at all. His wife and kids are starting to stay out of his way, just as he is simultaneously withdrawing more and more from them.

Logan also has been wrestling with a number of physical problems recently. His sleep is restless, with lots of tossing and turning, and he frequently has nightmares. He feels as if his eyesight is getting poorer, and he's definitely experiencing more headaches and more soreness in his neck and shoulders. He starts to tire now by late morning or early afternoon.

All of these problems Logan attributes to the longer hours he's been working, stooped over a computer. Some details, however, don't quite fit this explanation. For example, he comes to realize that his muscle soreness seems to get worse, not better, when he is walking outside in the brisk autumn air. He tells himself that maybe it's just because autumn is his least favorite season: he associates it with dying leaves and the end of sunny, outdoor fun.

Logan's wife finally convinces him to see a doctor for his complaints. The doctor finds no physical health problem, but he can tell that Logan is suffering from stress. The doctor advises him to take life more easily and gives him some pain medications to help alleviate his neck and shoulder soreness.

Logan is surprised to experience an unpleasant physical reaction to the medication, since he's taken it before without any side effects. Frustrated at the lack of much improvement in his health, he starts drinking a beer or two to relax before going to bed.

Logan's story manifests several key attributes of a person with a Wood constitution. Among them are a dark complexion; a strong, muscular, or stocky physique; and a fundamentally active, energetic nature. A tree (a basic Wood image) is symbolic of youthful vigor: the steady growth from a seedling into a fully mature specimen standing tall and pointing up into the air. Trees suggest a clear sense of direction in life; correspondingly, a Wood person tends to have not only a straight back, but also a facility at making plans and decisions.

When Wood people are living in an unhealthy or unbalanced manner, they start losing their vigor and sense of purpose. Instead, they easily become irritable, angry, and resentful, like a child with little tolerance for frustration. Just as a tree tends to be most healthy or vulnerable at the top, where new growth develops, so a Wood person tends to feel most alive—or most troubled—in the head, neck, shoulders, and upper back. This helps account for Logan's migraines and excessive soreness in the neck and shoulders.

Of all the weather elements in nature, the tree tends to be most susceptible to the wind—being either swayed, bent, splintered, or even uprooted by it. In a similar fashion, the Wood person may have a pronounced physical vulnerability to wind. This shows up in Logan, for example, in the way his neck and shoulders become even more sore when he walks outside in the brisk autumn wind.

Logan's problems can be treated in several different ways according to Chinese medical practices: both those that relate to people of all types and those that specifically address Wood-related problems. For example, in addition to working a lighter or more flexible schedule, Logan can recharge his energetic battery by taking a few minutes every two to three hours to do some of the meditation and Qigong exercises described in chapter 4. Even at work, he can periodically do one to two minutes of the very short exercises outlined in chapter 4. Another thing he can do is avoid going out in the night air, or if he does, he can wear a scarf to protect his neck and shoulders.

Logan also needs to pay closer attention to his diet. He probably started craving more sour (acidic) foods such as vinaigrette dressing and orange juice because his body was trying to regulate a Wood Qi imbalance. However, he is now overconsuming sour foods and needs to cut down on them so that he can achieve a better balance among all five food flavors: bitter, sweet, spicy, and salty as well as sour.

Because the Kidney nurtures the Liver (Water nurtures Wood, as explained in chapter 2), Logan also can help balance his Liver energy by eating salty foods (beneficial to the Kidney). In addition, he should eat foods that better balance hot and cold properties in his body—such as a hot sandwich for lunch instead of a cold salad. These issues and other dietary guidelines are discussed in chapter 4 and in the chapter 6 entries for individual health problems.

Logan's adverse reaction to medication also is related to his Liver condition. Because medications are metabolized in the liver, his Liver Qi imbalance makes them more difficult to process and more potentially upsetting. Overcoming the bad side effects of medications is discussed in chapter 7. Logan's consumption of alcohol puts an even greater burden on his liver.

Julie: The Fire Type

Logan works two offices down from Julie. You remember her— the laughing woman you met earlier. As annoying as her laugh can be to Logan, he prefers it to her door-slamming and wall-pounding. Julie's anger can be explosive!

Most of the time, however, Logan and Julie function well as a team: while Logan is good at making decisions, Julie is skilled at understanding the inner dynamics of a situation. Sometimes he's even attracted to her romantically, although he wonders if her reddish hue comes from too much makeup, and he doesn't like all the red clothes she wears.

What ultimately turns Logan off, however, is Julie's occasional indulgence in almost manic behavior, with little consideration of others around her. Many times when he's feeling an early-afternoon slump in energy, she'll burst into his office brimming with new ideas for this and that. She's generally quick in everything she does—walking, talking, eating, or going through a pile of paperwork—but sometimes she's almost frenzied.

Lately Julie has had to work harder, and the excess strain on her nerves has made her munch more than usual on her favorite bitter chocolate candy. While it was still summer and the weather was hot, she started feeling vague pains and muscle aches all over her body; but now that fall has arrived, those pains aren't quite as bad. Occasionally she feels her heart race, but she tries to ignore it by staying busy.

As you may have guessed, Julie is a Fire type. Think of all the physical and metaphorical qualities you can associate with fire, and you have a pretty good picture of her. Fire can provide illumination and warmth (as evidenced by Julie's ability to see into situations and, in turn, to be understanding), but it also can be explosive (as evidenced by her anger).

Above all, fire is energy. It stays active, and it moves quickly. Emotionally, a Fire type can function clearly and confidently, but he or she is also can go through great, agitated swings of passion and nervousness, fury and fatigue. Fire people are attracted to bitter or burned-tasting foods such as bitter chocolate, and their time of maximum energy is 11 A.M. to 3 P.M.—the energetic nadir for Wood people such as Logan. The organs associated with Fire are the Heart and Small Intestine. The Heart is the Emperor organ—the so-called House of Shen or Spirit, as well as the seat of emotions. The color for Fire is red, which is reflected in Julie's red complexion and her preference for red clothing. Fire also is associated with summer and with vulnerability to heat.

If Julie knew these things, she could keep herself a lot healthier and happier with the guidelines offered in this book. For starters, she could do some of the same meditations and exercises that would benefit Logan to calm down her nervousness and agitation.

Julie also needs to stop eating so much bitter food and to incorporate more of the other kinds of food into her diet. For example, Logan's vinaigrette dressing would be nurturing for her, since Wood nurtures Fire. To help relieve her heart palpitations, she should follow the recommendations in chapter 4 regarding foods that are good for the Heart, as well as some calming exercises in chapter 5.

Maria: The Earth Type

As it stands now, Julie simply suffers through her problems. When her mother, Maria, expresses concern about them, Julie characteristically snaps back, "I'm okay! Get off my back! I'm not a little girl anymore! I can take care of myself!" Maria, however, can't help worrying. A plump woman in her late forties, she's an Earth type, or, to put it in Western terms, a classic Earth Mother.

As an Earth type, Maria is essentially easygoing, kind, generous, and sympathetic—a real people-hugger—but also inclined to worry, or even obsess, when trouble looms. Unlike her daughter, she tends to do everything slowly. The one area where they cooperate beautifully is in sharing a box of chocolates: Maria takes all the sweet ones, and Julie takes all the bitter. In fact, Maria loves to eat. Her fleshy body, her attraction to late summer (harvest season), her large head, and her wide jaws are all traits associated with Earth people. Others include her short fingers, triangular-shaped nails, and a tendency to be most active between 7 A.M. and 11 A.M.

In recent weeks Maria has canceled plans with Julie several times because of a stomach ache, diarrhea, or fatigue. The organs associated with Earth are the Stomach and the Spleen/Pancreas, which makes the Earth person vulnerable to digestive disorders, especially after eating an excessive amount of sweet foods. The digestive system itself is very sensitive to dampness, both internal (fluid accumulation—e.g., due to edema) and external (rainy weather or damp living quarters). Such dampness also can cause a feeling of heaviness in the legs, which can be interpreted as fatigue.

If Julie were to use this book to help Maria, she would advise her to cut back on sweet foods (no doubt Julie also would stop tempting her with chocolates!). She would then assist her mother to work out a simple, easily managed diet plan based on chapters 4 and 6 that would help eliminate internal dampness and heal the digestive system. Before long Maria would start feeling healthier, less worrisome, and better able to cope with the sternness of her husband George.

George: The Metal Type

Maria's husband, George, is thrifty, organized, and independent by nature. He therefore finds it difficult to deal with Maria's comparative laxness and need for others. As a very rational, strong-willed person, he also can't truly empathize with Maria when she gets in one of her worrisome moods.

These characteristics indicate that George is a Metal person, and in fact he looks it. Tall and thin with square shoulders and angular features, he stands in sharp contrast to his soft, slightly overweight wife. Like other Metal people, he doesn't cry or otherwise show his emotions; but he is inclined toward sadness, and his voice does have a weepy quality. He coughs a lot early in the morning and has suffered from asthma since early childhood.

George also possesses many other Metal characteristics, including long fingers with rectangular nails, a tendency toward deliberate movements, a vulnerability to dryness, and a preference for spicy foods and the color white. The organs associated with Metal are the Lungs and the Large Intestine, and Metal people are inclined to develop respiratory disorders and bowel problems such as constipation. They favor autumn, and their time of maximum energy is 3 A.M.–7 A.M.

If Maria were familiar with this book, she would encourage George to use its relevant meditation, exercise, and diet guidelines to treat his early-morning phlegm and asthmatic symptoms. The book also could motivate and assist him to lead a more balanced life in terms of all Five Elements and, as a consequence, become less susceptible to sadness and more disposed to get along with others.

Max: The Water Type

One person in Julie's world who *does* seem familiar with Chinese medicine is Max—the man who shocked her with his pertinent advice at the party. Max is a Water type. It's physically apparent in his roundish face and body; short, puffy hands; crescent-moon-shaped fingernails; moany-groany voice; good hearing and balance; and strong bones and teeth.

Mentally and emotionally, Max's Water nature shows in his loyalty, sensitivity, and sympathy. He sometimes has difficulty understanding things; but at other times, he experiences sudden, almost psychic insights. When things are going well, he has ambition and willpower; when they're not, he tends to be fearful, suspicious, and in extreme cases, even paranoid.

The organs associated with Water are the Kidney and the Bladder, which accounts for Max's susceptibility to Kidney infections. He has a Water person's predilection toward black or navy-blue colors and salty foods (think of the ocean) and a special vulnerability to cold. His most energetic period of the day is between 3 P.M. and 7 P.M.

Some Elemental Observations

The five portraits you've just read give you a good working sense of the Five-Element types in their purest expression: Wood, Fire, Earth, Metal, and Water. In reality, most people are a composite of two or more types and therefore have a corresponding mix of characteristics and vulnerabilities that bear watching. For example, to evaluate the health of a person with a high number of Earth and Wood qualities, you would need to consider both Earth- and Wood-related health issues.

As a general rule, an exaggeration of a characteristic trait within a given elemental type may signal a health imbalance, but an even stronger indicator is the appearance of an uncharacteristic trait. For example, Fire people typically walk fast. When they walk more swiftly than usual, they may be suffering a health imbalance. However, an even more serious problem is suggested when they start walking more *slowly* than usual.

Now that you have a sense of the basic factors in Chinese health evaluation, you can begin observing yourself and others to detect possible patterns of health and illness that fit certain Yin-Yang and Five-Element patterns. This detection process becomes easier and easier, and more and more helpful, the more you apply it. Reading about various general therapies and specific treatments in the rest of this book will make the Yin-Yang and Five-Element patterns even more comprehensible and practical, and we'll start in the next chapter by examining how they relate to foods.

CHAPTER 4

Healthy Ways to Eat and Drink

One of the greatest benefits that Chinese medicine has to offer is a healthier approach to what, when, where, how, and how much we eat and drink, especially when we're sick. Based on centuries of effective experimentation in Chinese households—and bolstered by equally successful research and treatment by Chinese medical experts—this approach can be adopted in Western homes in a variety of ways that are surprisingly easy and fun to apply.

Western medicine, too, has provided us with a host of daily dietary recommendations. Among these recommendations, the most widely known and generally applicable are those that the USDA Food and Nutrition Board provides. We can use these very sensible guidelines along with Chinese ones to help guarantee that our diet is as healthy as possible.

Relying solely on the Western directives, however, leaves some critical gaps. Most do not take into account the possible effects of a food's freshness, flavor, temperature, and method of cooking on various systems in the body. Instead, there tends to be an overemphasis on calorie and fat intake, as befits a culture plagued by obesity and eating disorders and intent on quantifying anything and everything. Modern science is still baffled by these conditions and others relating to food because they haven't yet been adequately explained biochemically. Meanwhile, Chinese medicine has been addressing such problems successfully for centuries in its own, more holistic way.

Chapter 6 gives specific advice on what's healthiest to eat and drink during different kinds of illnesses. In this chapter we'll explore four basic principles that underlie the Chinese medical guidelines:

1. the Yin and Yang of food
2. the Five Elements in relation to food
3. the food-season relationship
4. food temperatures

In the course of this discussion, you can also pick up lots of other useful information, such as:

* how to prepare and serve food in the most favorable frame of mind and in the healthiest possible circumstances
* how to make simple and healthy changes in cooking processes
* how to relate what you eat to your element type or types and what you serve a sick family member to his or her element type or types
* how to replace processed foods with healthier natural foods in a manner that best suits you and your family

The Yin and Yang of Food

In chapter 3 you learned about Yin-Yang characteristics as they apply to a human being's physical, emotional, and spiritual constitution. Individual foods also have Yin and Yang qualities. You can, for example, balance an excess of Yin characteristics by eating foods with more Yang qualities, or treat an illness involving a Yin deficiency by eating foods with more Yin qualities.

Consider Alice, a woman who's been experiencing a variety of troubling, even alarming, symptoms for some time now. She has chronically dry skin. She often feels thirsty and consequently drinks a large amount of liquids during the day, though apparently not enough to slake her thirst altogether. At night she sweats during her sleep. She also tends to be constipated and urinates very little. Fortunately, she is mindful about her day-to-day health and lifestyle—something Chinese medicine encourages one to be. She notices that her symptoms tend to improve after she's eaten apples, and she recalls that on her worst day of symptoms, she ate handfuls of pistachio nuts and a seafood salad at dinner loaded with shrimp and lobster.

Alice contacts her doctor, but her symptoms don't add up to fit any Western medical diagnosis; they are too diffused throughout her body and not confined to any specific organ system. Chinese medicine, however, can identify her problem right away as a Yin deficiency. When there's not enough water (Yin) in the body, Yang symptoms such as dry skin or constipation become more prominent. Her reactions to certain foods also provide clues to her illness, as you will see later on.

Lately Alice's boyfriend, Jared, is also experiencing an odd assortment of symptoms. He's tired all the time. His hands and feet are often cold, and his skin seems paler and puffier than normal. Unlike Alice, he urinates a lot, especially at night. According to a Chinese medical evaluation of these symptoms, Jared suffers from a Yang deficiency—the opposite kind of problem from the one Alice has. He lacks "fire" in his constitution, so he's going through a period of excess water. Chinese medicine posits that the Kidney is the foundation of all the other organs. Therefore, Kidney Yin is the basis of all Yin in the body; Kidney Yang is the basis of all Yang. This means that any physical Yin and Yang symptoms basically reveal Kidney Yin and Kidney Yang states. Because the Kidney controls fluids in the body, Yin deficiencies tend to manifest themselves in symptoms of dryness; Yang deficiencies, in symptoms of wetness.

For more on Yin-Yang symptoms, and to help determine your own Yin-Yang state of being, see the chart on page 80.

Healing with foods follows the same Yin-Yang principle of strengthening what is deficient and minimizing what is excessed so that the opposites coexist in a state of harmony and balance. Strengthening foods are called tonics. When you are Yin-deficient, you need to eat more Yin Tonics and fewer Yang Tonics; when Yang-deficient, more Yang Tonics and fewer Yin Tonics.

Below are lists of both kinds of tonics. Note that these lists and others throughout the book feature foods and beverages that are commonly available in the West and that Western medical experts frequently include on their lists of healthy foods.

Yin Tonics

abalone	cantaloupes	duck
apples	cheeses	eggs (chicken)
asparagus	clams	figs
bananas	coconut milk	fungus (white)
barley	crab	grapes
beets	cuttlefish	honey
blackberries	dates	kidney beans

lemons

mandarin
    oranges

mangoes

microalgae
    (especially
    chlorella and
    spirulina)

millet

milk (cow)

mussels

oysters

peas

pears

pineapples

pomegranates

pork

rice

sardines

sea cucumbers

seaweed

shrimp

star fruit

string beans

sugar (white
    and cane)

tomatoes

tofu

walnuts

watermelons

wheat

wheat germ

yams

(*Note:* You can enhance the healing properties of dishes with
these foods by adding more liquid, such as by making stews,
soups, or porridges.)

Yang Tonics

chestnuts

cinnamon

cloves

dill seeds

fennel seeds

lobster

mandarin orange
    seeds (not pulp
    or juice)

oxtail

pistachio nuts

raspberries

star anise

strawberries

Yin-Yang: Excess and Deficiency Conditions

Excess Yang = Yin Deficiency	Excess Yin = Yang Deficiency
dryness: dry skin, throat, mouth	moist skin; edema
thirsty	not thirsty
constipation	loose stools
decreased urine	copious urine, enuresis
dry cough or thick sputum	moist cough, watery sputum
hypermetabolic symptoms: fast heart rate, nervousness; over a long period of time, body becomes thin and even wasted in extreme cases	hypometabolic symptoms: slowness, tendency toward weight gain
red complexion, red tongue, red cheeks, red eyes, sores in mouth, nosebleeds	pale complexion
feels hot, dislikes heat, likes cold	feels cold, likes warmth, dislikes cold
warm hands and feet; often sweaty; more spontaneous sweating	cold hands and feet; backache
heaviness or pain in the head	heaviness in lower part of the body
red rashes, hives	pale rashes
mentally more agitated, impatient; insomnia; irritable; excess thoughts	mentally sluggish
sexual dysfunction: decreased semen; premature ejaculation in men; menstrual disorders in women	sexual dysfunction: male impotence; female infertility
overall heat symptoms: easily excitable, loud	overall: fatigue, slow growth, slow movement; not excitable
underweight	overweight

Qi Tonics

Another form of Yang deficiency is general Qi deficiency, which can occur due to physical or emotional stress, chronic illness, improper diet, too much work, too much exercise, or aging beyond forty. The symptoms over several weeks or months are similar to those for Yang deficiency, only milder: fatigue (to the point of occasionally being too tired to talk), a lower-than-normal voice, a general feeling of weakness, a poor appetite, abdominal swelling, chronically soft stools, and frequent colds or infections. Fortunately, these foods can help alleviate a general Qi deficiency:

beef

bird's nest soup

bitter gourd
   seeds

cherries

chicken

coconut

dates (red and
   black)

eel

gingko

ginseng

goose

grapes

herring

honey

jackfruit

licorice

longan

lotus root powder

mackerel

octopus

pigeon (egg and
   meat)

potatoes (sweet
   and white)

rabbit

rice

shark's fin

shitake mush-
   rooms

squash

string beans
   (white)

sturgeon

sugar (rock)

tofu

Blood Tonics

Because Qi is the driving force for Blood, a Qi deficiency is often accompanied by a Blood deficiency. The latter might be aggravated by any bleeding condition, such as menstruation, nosebleeds, or bleeding from a polyp or tumor. The most common Western diagnosis of this kind of deficiency is anemia, and its symptoms include dizziness, palpitations, nervousness, a pale complexion, numbness in the hands and feet, and, in women, a lightening of the menstrual flow. The Heart's association with the Spirit means that there also may be an inability to concentrate as well as insomnia and forgetfulness. These foods can help:

beef	liver (beef and pork)	oxtail
cuttlefish		oysters
eggs (chicken)	longan	palm seed
grapes	milk (human breast)	sea cucumber
ham		spinach
lichi nuts	octopus	

The Tonics: A Little Goes a Long Way

The Yin Tonics, Yang Tonics, Qi Tonics, and Blood Tonics are good for general strengthening of their respective deficiencies. You can evaluate such deficiencies in yourself and others by using the chart on page 80 and the various symptom lists above. You can then treat them by incorporating more of the appropriate tonics into your day-to-day diet.

Always remember, however, that the key to healing lies in moderation. The tonics are considered medicines; as with Western medicines, it's not healthy to overdose. Step-by-step change is less jarring to body systems, so work toward minor adjustments, not radical revisions.

Eating tonic foods is also not advisable during the course of an active infection. There is a famous expression in Chinese medicine about "not trapping the burglar." When a burglar is in your house, you have two basic options. First, there's the "trapping" one—that is, trying to kill the burglar, in which case you may succeed and be left to deal with the mess, both physically and emotionally; or you may fail and be left to deal with the enraged burglar. The second option is, overall, the more sensible one: scaring the burglar away, preferably before he gets all the loot.

In medical terms, the infection is the burglar. Taking tonic foods represents the aggressive, confrontational first option, which can inadvertently strengthen the burglar and create more problems than you bargained for. "Not trapping the burglar" means employing the second kind of option: getting rid of the infection *before* strengthening the body. For example, you want to help your body to sweat during an infection so that Qi can circulate and drive out the "impurity" through the pores. Then you can take Qi and Blood Tonics to help your weakened but now "pure" body recover.

Finally, one last warning: avoid too many tonic foods when there's a digestive problem. It's hard to benefit from such foods anyway if you can't digest them properly or if you vomit them back out. Instead, follow the dietary guidelines in chapter 6 for specific digestive ailments. Also, see the discussion in chapter 5 about tonifying your Spleen/Pancreas.

Now that you have reviewed the basics of Yin-Yang–related body states, what do you do if you can't decide whether a given problem represents a Yin deficiency, a Yang deficiency, a Blood deficiency, or a Qi deficiency? You go a step farther, to explore how the Five Elements factor into health, illness, and diet.

Food and the Five Elements

In chapter 2 you discovered that the Five Elements—Wood, Fire, Earth, Metal, and Water—correspond to the body systems and the seasons. In chapter 3 you figured out which of the Five Elements fit your overall physical, mental, emotional, and spiritual constitution, and you learned how to evaluate other people to find out their major elemental type or types. It's time to fill in another piece of the picture: how the Five Elements of food relate to different body systems, seasons, and constitutional types.

This additional perspective makes it all the clearer how Chinese medicine works to integrate you more naturally and healthfully with the universe as a whole. At the same time, properly administrated according to the guidelines in this book, Chinese medicine doesn't interfere with any Western medical regimen you may be following, either to maintain day-to-day general health or to treat a specific condition. In fact, the two approaches complement each other.

According to Five-Element theory, foods are classified according to their taste (or flavor) and their season of predominance, each of which helps determine their healing value for a particular body system and for a particular time of year. A table of correspondences occurs on page 85.

Let's begin with the first major question relating to food that the table raises: What does it mean that a certain influences a particular Yin-Yang combination of organs?

Throughout the ages, Chinese physicians have noticed that people are healthier when their diet balances the five basic flavors listed above. Chinese physicians also have learned that when the diet features a deficiency in or an excess of a certain flavor, a particular organ system suffers or weakens. When a moderate amount of that flavor is added to the diet, that system becomes healthier. For example, when there is not enough or

The Five Elements: Food Tastes and Other Correspondences

Element	Taste	Organs	Time of Year
Wood	Sour	Liver and Gallbladder	Spring
Fire	Bitter	Heart and Small Intestine	Summer
Earth	Sweet	Spleen/Pancreas and Stomach	Late Summer
Metal	Pungent/ Spicy	Lung and Large Intestine	Autumn
Water	Salty	Kidney and Bladder	Winter

too much consumption of sour-flavored food, the Liver and the Gallbladder are prone to become unbalanced and to manifest symptoms of illness, and so on.

In addition, Chinese experts have established that each person has a particularly vulnerable organ system and therefore an especially strong reaction to a certain taste, according to his or her major elemental type or types. For example, let's take Julie, the Fire type from chapter 3. The flavor corresponding to Fire is bitter, and the organs are the Heart and Small Intestine. She ate a lot of bitter chocolate and developed heart palpitations. Her coworker Logan, a Wood type, could have eaten the same amount of bitter chocolate and not had as serious a Heart reaction precisely because he is not, like Julie, a Fire type. Her extra-fine attunement to the bitter flavor makes her predisposed to develop Heart imbalances more easily based on the amount of bitter food she eats—or doesn't eat.

The five flavors should be fairly well balanced in the diet of a healthy person. No precise measurement is required, and you don't need to make sure that one-fifth of your diet consists of each element. Instead, it's a matter of becoming more aware of your diet-related tendencies.

For example, is a certain taste very rare in your diet? If so, it's wise to increase your intake of that taste regularly. One way you can do this is to pick out two or three foods with that taste that you're willing to eat more often. Is another taste very prominent in your diet? If so, it's wise to cut down on your consumption of foods with that taste.

The sweet flavor tends to predominate in most people's diet because most natural foods—including grains, vegetables, nuts, seeds, and fruits—have this taste. A reasonable predominance, however, is compatible with human physiology, because the digestive organs (the Spleen/Pancreas and the Stomach) are related to Earth and, therefore, sweetness.

Regrettably, many foods made today contain an overabundance of artificial sweeteners. Typical examples are soda, juice, tea drinks, candies, cookies, and cakes. Artificial flavors should be added only in small amounts to provide a balance of five flavors: for example, extra salt can be added if there's a deficiency of salty foods in the diet.

For more general guidelines, let's look at each flavor and the major organ associated with it.

Sour: Liver (Wood)

Sour is a Yin flavor and tends to cause contraction, which has an astringent effect on body fluids and energy. It enters the Liver and helps with digesting rich, greasy, fatty, and high-cholesterol foods. The taste derives from a great variety of acids, including citric, tannic, and ascorbic (vitamin C). It's the least common taste in the Western diet.

The most purely sour flavors occur in black and green teas and blackberry leaves. Other sour foods are hawthorn berries, lemons, limes, pickles, rose hips, sauerkraut, sour apples (crab-apples), and sour plums. Some foods feature a combination of sour taste and some other taste, such as:

- sour and bitter: vinegar
- sour and pungent/spicy: leeks
- sour and sweet: apples, blackberries, cheese, grapes, huckle-berries, mangoes, olives, raspberries, sourdough bread, tan-gerines, tomatoes, and yogurt

Because Wood nurtures Fire, a sour taste can help with certain Heart-Mind conditions, such as an inability to concentrate or a sense of being scattered. It also can be used sparingly in cases of arthritis, tendonitis, dry skin, or constipation. Alternatively, it should be avoided or decreased when there's a Spleen/Pancreas or Stomach deficiency, since Wood controls Earth.

To tonify your Liver, you need to consume almost equal amounts of salty and sour foods, with proportionately fewer pungent/spicy ones. The salt flavor helps because Water nurtures Wood. The pungent/spicy flavor is problematic because Metal destroys Wood.

Bitter: Heart (Fire)

Bitter is a Yin flavor, a cooling one that moves Qi downward in the body. A moderate amount of bitter foods can reduce excess conditions such as loudness, a red complexion, and aggressiveness, but too much sometimes can bring about the opposite effect. The bitter flavor also can reduce fever, clear heat (e.g., from eating too many rich foods), bring about dryness, and lower blood pressure (e.g., celery often is recommended for people with high blood pressure).

Bitter foods include most medications as well as alfalfa, bitter melon, burdock leaf or root, chamomile, dandelion leaf or root, echinacea, hops, romaine lettuce, rye, and valerian. Other foods feature a combination of bitter taste and some other taste, such as:

- bitter and pungent/spicy: citrus peel (also sweet), radish leaves, scallions, turnips (also sweet), and white pepper
- bitter and sweet: asparagus, bitter chocolate, celery, lettuce, papaya, quinoa
- bitter and sour: vinegar

Many people find a bitter taste too harsh and therefore incorporate it into their diet by combining it with naturally sweet foods—see the following sections, "Sweet: Spleen/Pancreas (Earth)."

A bitter taste also combats edema and lethargy and benefits people who tend to be slow-moving or overweight. Because Fire nurtures Earth, bitter foods can be used sparingly to bolster Spleen/Pancreas deficiencies. They should also be used sparingly with people who tend to be cold, weak, or dry. Because Fire controls Metal, people who have excess Lung-related symptoms, such as pneumonia with fever and yellow phlegm, should minimize their intake of bitter foods.

Sweet: Spleen/Pancreas (Earth)

Sweet is a Yang flavor that generally has a warming effect and moves Qi upward and outward through the skin. Sweet builds tissues and fluids—the Yin of the body—and therefore also strengthens Yin deficiencies. It's the most common flavor in foods and can be subdivided into two categories: full sweet foods, which are more tonifying and strengthening; and empty sweet foods, which are more cleansing and cooling.

The most important sweet foods are all of the grains. Carbohydrates such as grains are the mainstay of most diets. They break down into glucose (sugar), which feeds the brain and provides energy. Other sweet foods include all of the legumes (beans, peas, and lentils), most meats, and most dairy products. In addition, there are the following sweet foods, listed by food group and, if relevant, subgroups combining sweet with another flavor:

- fruit: apples, apricots, cherries, dates, figs, papayas
- sweet and sour fruit: grapes, grapefruit, olives, peaches, strawberries, tomatoes
- vegetables: beets, button mushrooms, carrots, chard, cucumbers, eggplant, peas, potatoes, shiitake mushrooms, squash, sweet potatoes, yams
- sweet and pungent/spicy vegetables: cabbages, spearmint
- sweet and bitter vegetables: celery, lettuce
- nuts and seeds: almonds, chestnuts, coconuts, sesame seeds and oil, pine nuts, sunflower seeds, walnuts
- sweeteners: barley malt, molasses, rice syrup, whole sugar
  Sweet and pungent/spicy sweetener: honey. (*Note:* Honey may be helpful in drying up mucus conditions but should not be used in people who tend to be dry and suffer deficiencies or who are nervous or thin. It has a drying effect on the body after digestion.)

To tonify your Spleen/Pancreas when they're experiencing health problems, you need to have almost equal amounts of sweet and bitter foods in your diet, with proportionately fewer sour foods. This is because Fire (bitter) nurtures Earth, while Wood (sour) destroys it.

Because Earth nurtures Metal in particular, naturally sweet foods can assist the Lungs, especially during a state of deficiency. Naturally sweet foods also are good for individuals who are somehow physiologically deficient: dry, cold, nervous, thin, or weak. Aggressive, angry, or impatient people can benefit from the retarding effect of the sweet flavor. In this kind of situation, extra consumption of wheat, rice, and oats often helps.

Sweet foods should be taken sparingly by people who are overweight or who have mucus or other "dampness" symptoms. For all individuals, but especially these people, it is important to chew carbohydrates and other sweet foods thoroughly. When the salivary enzymes in the mouth break down the foods, the digestive organs don't have to work as hard. Excess sweets weaken not only the Spleen/Pancreas but also the Lungs and the Kidneys.

Pungent/Spicy: Lung (Metal)

This flavor has Yang qualities. It warms the body, assists the circulation of Qi and Blood, stimulates the digestive process, disperses mucus, and enters the Lungs. The primary Lung conditions it can help alleviate are related to cough and mucus production, such as the common cold, bronchitis, and asthma.

Pungent/spicy foods are divided into the following categories depending on their effect (some foods appear in more than one category):

- diaphoretic (sweat-causing): cayenne, chamomile, elder flower, garlic, mint, scallion
  (*Note:* These foods induce beneficial sweating during a common cold or other, similar situations.)
- warming (cannot be used with fever): anise, basil, cayenne, cinnamon (bark and branch), cloves, dill, fennel, garlic, ginger root (fresh and dried), horseradish, mustard greens, nutmeg, onions (all kinds), pepper (black and all hot), rosemary, scallion, spearmint
  (*Note:* Cinnamon and dried ginger can provide warmth for a long period of time and overcome signs of coldness.)
- cooling (can be used with fever): elder flowers, marjoram, peppermint, radish leaves, white pepper
- neutral: taro, turnip
- seed: anise, caraway, coriander, cumin, dill, fennel
  (*Note:* These seeds relax the nervous system and improve digestion. They're especially beneficial for people who are

dry and thin or who tend toward nervousness and restlessness.)
- root: ginger, onion (cooked), horseradish, peppercorn (black)
  (*Note:* These roots promote general stability and smooth circulation of energy.)
  extremely hot spicy: cayenne, fresh ginger, and black pepper as well as hot green and red peppers
  (*Note:* The warming effect is short-lasting. It changes to a cooling effect after thirty minutes.)

The medicinal potency of pungent/spicy foods can be diminished by cooking.

To tonify your Lungs, you need to eat almost equal amounts of sweet foods (Earth nurtures Metal) and pungent/spicy foods, with proportionately fewer bitter foods (Fire destroys Metal). Because Metal nurtures Water, cautious consumption of pungent/spicy foods (avoiding excess) can help people with a Kidney Yang deficiency who are manifesting cold symptoms. Pungent/spicy foods also should be consumed sparingly in dry and heat conditions and, since Metal controls Wood, in cases of Liver disorder.

Salt: Kidney (Water)

Salt is a Yin flavor and tends to cool, moisten, and detoxify the body, increase appetite, and improve digestion. It is beneficial in conditions of dryness (e.g., gargling with salt water is advisable for sore throat; and brushing the teeth with fine salt, for mild gum inflammations).

Major salty foods are salt itself and seaweed (such as kelp). Other substantially salty foods are gomasio (sesame salt), miso, pickles, and soy sauce. Barley and millet are primarily sweet foods, but they also have salty qualities.

To tonify your Kidneys, you need to consume equal amounts

of salt and pungent/spicy foods (Metal nurtures Water), with proportionately fewer sweet foods (Earth destroys Water). Be cautious about increasing salt intake in cases of excess fluid (such as edema), high blood pressure, a kidney disorder where kidney function is impaired, or an overweight body. Because Water controls Fire, excess salt also can have an adverse effect on the Heart.

The Food-Season Relationship

Let's now look at how the Five Elements are linked with the five seasons of weather and how that link helps determine the health value of what we eat. The main point to keep in mind is that the more we can attune our diet to the changes in the seasons, the more in harmony with nature we'll be, which translates into better health. It's also important to include each of the five flavors in your diet regardless of the season. However, the recommended proportion changes from season to season, as you will see in a moment.

It's especially important to consider the Five-Elements system when you have a particular, internal imbalance that's causing—or that may cause—illness. The seasonal dietary guidelines you're about to review are general recommendations for all of us to follow as we go through the year, in order to stay in proper, healthy rhythm with Nature. I'll briefly review each element-season correspondence individually.

Wood: Spring

Spring represents youth, renewal, and growth, like a tree ascending into the sky. A good diet during Spring reflects all of these characteristics. It's a time to eat lots of naturally sweet foods (Earth-related); green, leafy foods; sprouts and seeds; and raw or tender, young vegetables, such as baby carrots and small beets. Simultaneously the other kinds of tastes should also be represented in the diet to some degree.

Spring has left Winter, so it's the season to limit intake of salty foods (Winter-related). Because Wood is associated with the Liver, it's also advisable to cut down on Liver-taxing items such as fat, greasy foods; chemicals (e.g., medications are metabolized in the Liver); alcohol (young drinkers suffer more because of the Wood-youth link); and processed foods. Some experts believe that "spring fever" is related to ingesting seasonally inappropriate foods such as greasy and fattening ones that convert into heat and, therefore, fever. Because Metal controls Wood, pungent/spicy foods can be used to cleanse or detoxify the body (comparable to Western healers prescribing a week-long dose of raw onions and garlic to rid the body of parasites).

Chinese doctors often suggest using pungent/spicy herbs and seeds for cooking in the Spring, including basil, bay leaf, caraway, dill, fennel, marjoram, and rosemary. During this season, food is best cooked for a shorter time, but at a higher temperature. The preferred methods include stir-frying, sautéing with just a small amount of oil (to avoid Liver harm), and steaming or simmering lightly. A Spring diet also needs to be balanced with more active physical exercise.

Fire: Summer

Among all the elements, Fire is the most Yang and therefore is associated with the hottest season, Summer. It's a time of maturation, passion, and joy when it's good to get outdoors a lot: to walk, camp, garden, lie in the sun, or involve ourselves in community affairs.

Summer is also the time to eat brightly colored fruits, vegetables, and flowers and to enjoy equally colorful tablecloths, napkins, and floral arrangements. Eat fresh, locally grown foods—as opposed to foods from far-off places—to achieve more harmony with your immediate environment. For example, if you live in the Midwest, avoid tropical fruits in favor of watermelons and apples.

Food preparation should take as little time as possible: cook quickly using high heat. Because Water controls Fire, use salty foods sparingly, but make sure there is some degree of salty taste as well as sour and bitter tastes in your diet. Drink plenty of water so you don't get dehydrated.

Pungent/spicy foods sometimes can be beneficial because they trigger sweating: for example, cayenne, ginger (fresh, not dried), horseradish, and pepper (black as well as red and green hot peppers). The principle here is to bring the body into harmony with the temperature of the environment. The hotness of the food causes a dispersal of body heat through the pores, so that the skin temperature more closely approximates the hot Summer temperature and, accordingly, the body feels more comfortable. This is why countries in the tropics frequently have very spicy cuisine. Moderation is important: if you eat too many hot, spicy foods in the Summer, you can lose too much internal heat, leaving your body in a colder-than-healthy state as you enter Autumn and Winter.

Contrary to modern Western practice, ice-cold drinks or foods are not recommended even during the hottest Summer days. Putting such foods into the Stomach is like giving it a shock: it contracts, and the digestive process slows down. In addition, the pores contract so they don't sweat, resulting ultimately in a more uncomfortable feeling. The same sort of shock occurs when you move quickly from the hot outside air into a very cold, air-conditioned room.

A healthier kind of coolness can be achieved on hot summer days by sitting in the shade and eating the right foods, such as salads with sprouts, alfalfa, and cucumbers; vegetables such as tofu; fruits such as watermelons, apples, and lemons; and drinks such as chrysanthemum, mint, and chamomile teas. In general, eat light foods and avoid heavy ones such as meat, eggs, and an overabundance of grains, nuts, and seeds.

Earth: Late Summer

This is approximately the last month of Summer, when there tends to be the most balanced weather—not too hot, not too cold. It's the time of harvest and transition from Yang (growth) to Yin (rest). Choose to slow down and do things in moderation. Center yourself with meditation and engage in physical, mental, and spiritual activities that make you feel more in tune with Mother Earth.

The color for Earth is yellow, and the flavor is sweet. This suggests more consumption of foods such as carrots, yellow corn, and yellow squash. Other good, mostly round-shaped foods that tend to center us are apricots, cabbage, cantaloupe, chestnuts, filberts, garbanzo beans, millet, peas, rice, soybeans, string beans, sweet potatoes, sweet rice, and tofu.

Foods need to be seasoned mildly, as opposed to the spicier taste of Summer. Late Summer foods should be cooked at a moderate temperature, whether baked, sautéed, stewed, or steamed. Serve simple dishes instead of elaborately prepared ones. All of these measures will help you prepare for the transition between Summer (Yang) and Autumn/Winter (Yin).

Metal: Autumn

Autumn begins the Yin time of year, a season for pulling inward and slowing down. It's also a time to plan for the Winter, Metal being associated with organization. Because Metal is connected with the Lungs, you need to give more attention to the fragrance of food. Let it cook on lower heat for a longer time so the smell permeates the kitchen and stimulates the appetite.

Autumn foods and cooking need to focus on supplying greater energy. Concentrated foods and roots thicken the blood for cooler weather. Because Metal is linked with dryness (dry skin or throat, or a thin body type with chronic dryness), eat foods that tend to moisten the body: almonds, apples, barley, barley malt, clams, crabs, dairy products, eggs, fungus (black and white), herring, honey (cooked), millet, mussels, oysters, peanuts, pears, persimmons, pine nuts, pork, rice syrup, seaweed, sesame seeds, spinach, and soybean products, including soy milk and tofu. Use a little salt in cooking. Consume sour and bitter tastes sparingly. Also be cautious with spices, especially strong ones such as cayenne.

Water: Winter

Winter is the opposite of Summer, as Water is the opposite of Fire. During Winter we become more Yin and need more rest as the days grow shorter. Just like hibernating animals, we need to keep the inside of our body warm, while contracting our pores to keep our skin cool so that we harmonize with the outside environment. It's a season to store up food and to gain a little weight that can be burned off the following Summer.

In Winter, warm, hearty soups with a little added salt are the perfect meals. Don't put in too much water, because an excess can weaken body systems, and cook the mixture at a low temperature for a long time. Unless salt is not advisable for medical reasons (such as a Kidney disorder or high blood pressure), increase your intake of salty, Kidney-nourishing foods such as barley, millet, miso, seaweed, salt, and soy sauce. To nourish the Heart and preserve joyfulness, these salty foods need to be counterbalanced with some bitter ones. It's also advisable to eat more Warm foods in the Winter (see the Warm food list on page 99).

Food Temperatures

Alan can't believe how quickly the weather has changed! Only last week he was walking around in shorts enjoying one bright, sunny day after another. All this week it's been rainy and cold. "I guess fall has arrived," he mutters, pulling a warm sweater out of his closet. He also grabs a box of cough drops from his medicine chest, knowing that he tends to develop a cough when the cold weather starts. At lunch he skips his usual yogurt because his doctor advised him that dairy products cause extra phlegm.

Most of us, like Alan, instinctively reach for warmer clothes when the weather gets cold. At the same time, we may also perform various cold-weather-related health rituals that we've learned from experience or been advised to do by others. Many of these are very sensible practices promoted by Western medicine, such as humidifying overly heated air and avoiding abrupt transitions from one extreme temperature to another. Few of us, however, pay attention to what our *internal* temperature may be, or care for it so automatically.

Just as the temperature outdoors can be hot or cold, warm or cool, so can the temperature inside our bodies. In addition, since we are part of the natural world, our internal temperature needs to be in harmony with the external temperature of Nature for us to stay healthy. Among other things, this means that our skin should feel healthily and comfortably warm during the Summer and cool during the Winter.

We also need to maintain a homeostatic temperature within our body so that all systems can function well with each other and within the natural world as a whole. For example, if our body is too cold internally on a hot day, we unfortunately need to absorb so much warmth from the sun that we aren't able to sweat to achieve a healthy, comfortable skin temperature. If our body's too hot on such a day, the skin becomes even hotter than the outdoors, which is just as unhealthy and uncomfortable.

According to Western medicine, body temperature changes are due to metabolism. The ideal norm for most body processes is 98.6 degrees Fahrenheit. A fever (higher temperature) is a sign of disease, and it's treated by taking tepid baths or medications. A lower-than-normal temperature indicates a potentially more serious disturbance, such as chronic illnesses, cancer, or exposure to very cold weather.

Chinese medicine also considers a measurable change in body temperature to be a signal of disorder. However, the Chinese also believe that subtler, less measurable temperature changes can indicate problems such as Qi imbalances. For example, a person can have a so-called Cold condition (not to be confused with the common cold) that manifests itself in having cold hands and feet or in feeling cold, even though the body temperature measures 98.6 degrees.

Because Qi is energy, and energy is warmth, a harmonious and well-balanced Qi flow should provide even temperature throughout the body—to the organs as well as to every millimeter of skin, from the trunk to the tips of the fingers. If it doesn't, there is bound to be some sort of evidence, such as a cold spot. The situation is analogous to the flow of blood. If the tiniest, pinpoint area on the skin has abnormal blood flow, that area will change color, producing red or purple dots known in Western medicine as petechiae.

Abnormal Qi flow cannot be visualized or measured in lab tests, but it can be experienced subjectively. Even when it isn't, it can be felt by a qualified examiner, simply through touching the upper and lower extremities or by probing the chest and upper and lower abdomen (called the Three Burners in Chinese medicine) for slight changes in skin temperature.

Our inner body temperature is greatly influenced by foods, both in making us go out of balance and in bringing us back into balance. This is because foods have thermoregulatory properties—that is, specific effects on our Qi flow that affect our body temperature. These properties are classified as follows:

- Hot: Yang foods that direct energy and fluid upward and outward to the skin; for example, beets, brussels sprouts, cinnamon, lamb, peaches, pepper (black, white, cayenne)
- Warm: similar to hot foods but milder in effect; for example, asparagus, chicken, peanuts, red wine, squash
- Cool: Yin foods that direct energy and fluid downward and inward so that the upper part of the body and the skin are cold; for example, barley, eggplant, pork, strawberries, tofu
- Cold: similar to cool foods but with stronger effect: for example, apples, celery, cottage cheese, mussels, salt.

Food Temperatures: Basic Guidelines

Here are various general points relating to the temperatures of foods:

- Plants that take a long time to grow (such as carrots and cabbages, which require six months) are more warming than those grown more quickly (such as lettuce and radishes).
- Chemically fertilized fruits and vegetables, which are stimulated to grow quickly, are generally more cooling than their organically raised counterparts.
- Foods with blue, green, or purple colors are generally more cooling than similar foods that are red, orange, or yellow (e.g., a green apple is more cooling than a red one).

The following are general guidelines relating to the effects of preparation and cooking on the temperatures of foods:

- When food is broken down by cutting, chopping, or grinding, more Qi and heat is released when they are eaten. This follows the basic Western physics principle that more heat exchange occurs with more surface area.
- Heating foods accomplishes two purposes: first, the external heat imparts more energy to the foods; second, heat helps break down food structure so that more nutrients are made available.
- Moderate cooking results in losing relatively few nutrients.
- Cooking methods that involve more cooking time, higher temperatures or pressure, more dryness, and/or more air circulation (e.g., convection-oven cooking) impart more warming qualities to food.
- Cooking for a long time on low heat is more warming than cooking for a short time on high heat.
- Among cooking methods, the usual order from most warming to least is: deep-frying or tempura, baking, stir-frying, sautéing, pressure cooking, simmering, steaming, and waterless cooking to below the boiling point. "Heatless" methods of breaking down food in progressively more cooling order are: fermenting, marinating, and sprouting.
- The cooking fuel affects the amount and quality of energy available in the cooked food. Electricity produces the lowest results and is not recommended for weak people. Microwave cooking damages the molecular structure of food and diminishes the Qi energy.
- In general, eating raw foods has a more cooling effect on the body than eating cooked foods, so that more of our existing Qi is required for digestion, leaving less Qi for other physiologic functions, both physical and mental.

Eating as a Healing Exercise

Healthy eating is more than just a digestive act. It is an experience involving all of our sensory organs: eyes, ears, nose, and skin as well as tongue. The major cuisines of the world—Eastern and Western—take great care in the presentation of food not just because it's a *nice* thing to do but also because it's a *healing* thing to do. It encourages us to value food, eat it more attentively, digest it more smoothly, and allow its nourishing properties—including temperature—to work more effectively.

When you eat food or serve it to others, bear these facts in mind, and do all you can to render the experience pleasant and soothing to every sense. Reserve plenty of time and space for relaxed, uninterrupted dining. Make the food and the table attractive. Play soft music and engage in easy, nonstressful conversation with other diners. Don't rush from eating to performing strenuous physical or mental work.

Also remember that chewing is a very important part of eating. In Western terms, enzymes in the saliva help to break down food. In Chinese terms, saliva is a "golden, precious fluid" that imparts warmth to food. Both West and East advocate chewing your food thoroughly.

Other guidelines on proper eating are offered in chapter 6, on an illness-by-illness basis. For a good, representative example with broad application to health problems, see the entry "Abdominal Pain."

Keep in mind that a well-balanced diet consists of the right amounts of hot, warm, cool, and cold foods. Too many hot or warm foods and too few cool or cold foods can lead to an excess Heat (or excess Yang) condition. Among the possible symptoms are dry mouth, constipation, thirst, red face, aversion to heat, sweaty palms, red rashes, a faster heart rate, and nervousness. Among the treatments for excess Heat are eating fewer hot or warm foods and more cool or cold foods; drinking more liquids; and reducing stress. Symptoms and treatments relating to specific health problems that involve excess Heat (Yang) are discussed in chapter 6 on an illness-by-illness basis.

The opposite condition, arising from eating too few hot or warm foods and too many cool or cold foods, is an excess Cold (excess Yin) condition. Among the symptoms may be chill sensations, copious urine, watery stools, increased fear, white complexion, aversion to cold, difficulty in moving, and so on. Among the treatments for excess Cold are eating more hot or warm foods and fewer cool or cold foods, and avoiding raw or microwaved foods. Again, the entries in chapter 6 cover specific symptoms and treatments of excess Cold (Yin) as it's associated with individual health problems.

We've covered a lot of ground in this chapter, and you may want to consult it again and again as you use the entries in chapter 6 to treat different illnesses with different kinds of food-related issues. Meanwhile, you can apply the information in this chapter by itself toward making small, beneficial modifications in the meals you eat and serve to others.

For example, be aware of whether you or others may benefit from more Yin Tonics or, alternatively, from more Yang Tonics. If you know that you have or someone else has problems with a particular organ system, put into practice some of the relevant advice in the "Food and the Five Elements" and "Food Temperatures" sections in this chapter. Strive in whatever ways you can to achieve a more balanced diet in all respects—according to Yin-Yang, the Five Elements, and food temperatures. And eat more of what's in season to help ensure that you're in harmony with Nature.

CHAPTER 5

Minutes a Day for Peace and Well-being

Besides enabling us to recover from illness, remain healthy, and live longer, Chinese medicine helps us to enjoy a high quality of life—not only physically, but emotionally and spiritually as well. We can go a long way toward achieving all four objectives just by doing a few simple healing activities each day. When combined with the kinds of exercises recommended by Western medicine (e.g., walking at least forty-five minutes at a time, three days a week, to keep the cardiovascular system in shape), they can be all the more effective.

This chapter offers some of the most effective Chinese healing that I've learned from Qigong (pronounced "chee-GONG") masters from all over the world, including Dr. Effie Chow of the United States, chair of the World Congress on Qigong. These activities are organized into seven groups:

- *good posture activity:* a simple technique for making sure your posture promotes healthy breathing and movement throughout each day
- *easy breathing activities:* deep abdominal breathing as well as various breathing cycles to sharpen awareness of different body systems
- *gentle cleansing and Qi-strengthening movements:* simple movements to cleanse the body of toxins and tonify Qi energy
- *meditations:* various practices aimed at clearing the mind, calming the body, and restoring the spirit
- *movement activities:* basic exercises derived from the Chinese arts of Qigong and Tai Chi (pronounced "tie-CHEE") to enhance body flexibility and control, to maintain health, and to relieve stress
- *soothing massages:* self- and partner-administered massage techniques for improving energy flow, increasing body consciousness, and alleviating tension
- *healing sound activities:* "singing" a variety of strong musical tones that create beneficial vibrations in different body systems

A major stumbling block for many people regarding any kind of fitness routine is the time/energy factor. It's a complaint I hear constantly from patients, in a host of different forms: "I'm too busy to exercise!" "My schedule's too crazy!" "When do I ever have five minutes at a time to call my own?" "Whenever I do get the time to work out, I'm too exhausted!"

If you've ever said something like this to yourself, then you'll especially appreciate the kind of "routines," "exercises," or "workouts" described in this chapter. First of all, they're exceptionally easy and refreshing. Second, they're quick. Depending on your schedule and preference, you can do all the relevant activities in a single, twenty-minute block of time, or you can do them individually at scattered moments throughout the day. Each takes only several seconds to a few minutes to do, depending on the activity, and many of them can be done wherever you happen to be: at home or at work, outdoors or indoors, even in a car.

Each activity is also easy to teach to others and fun to do with them whenever the opportunity presents itself. But you can start by yourself right now!

Good Posture

Carol just couldn't get comfortable. Her chair seemed too low for her computer. Her wrists and arms, as well as her lower back, were sore at the end of the day. She started doing some breathing exercises that a friend recommended. They helped somewhat, but did not give her much relief when she was actually sitting at her computer. Her doctor gave her a prescription for an ergonomic chair—one that "fits" her body type and most common working position. Her symptoms, however, persisted, and she decided to consult an acupuncturist.

When Carol came to me, I noticed that she sat slouched over, both in her chair and on the examining table. She told me she meditated regularly, and when I asked her to sit in her meditation position, I saw that her abdomen was crunched into a fold. I knew then why her breathing exercises (and, for that matter, her meditation and her ergonomic chair) weren't working as well as they should. The problem was her posture.

Proper posture is critically important to healthy breathing. Be sure to check your posture from time to time while you've engaged in *any* endeavor—sitting, standing, walking, or meditating—as well as whenever you're about to do a special breathing activity. Poor posture can affect not only our muscles and bones (the soreness Carol experienced) but also our Qi, or energy balance, which, in turn, influences our emotions and our ability to manage stress.

Here is a simplified version of Dr. Chow's well-known "Silver Thread" technique for achieving proper posture:

1. Hold your head in line with your trunk so that from a side view the ears are over the shoulders, which are pulled back instead of slouched toward the front.

2. Imagine a silver thread lifting you upward from the tailbone through the spine and through the DU 20 point at the top of your head. Locate this point by placing your thumbs on the tips of your ears and bringing your third fingers to the top of your head; let the fingertips touch in the middle of your head at a point where a line drawn from your nose and a line connecting the tips of the ears would intersect. It's also called the Hundred Meeting, or Bai Hui, point because it's where all the Yang energies in the body meet.

3. Feel the stretch of the spine caused by the pull of the thread, while keeping the shoulders back and down (you can grasp your hands behind your back and stretch to pull your shoulders into the right position). Let everything else hang loosely around the silver thread so you are in a relaxed, upright posture. Keep your body still and calm.

4. Visualize another silver thread pulling you forward from the Dantian (or "Seat of Life") point, located two inches below the navel and one inch inward. As the thread pulls, it should tilt your pelvis slightly, so your upper torso fits directly over the pelvis.

To maintain good posture whenever you are walking, hold the knees slightly flexed, not locked, and land with the balls of the feet on the ground instead of either the toes or the heels. When you're sitting, avoid sliding or slumping down into the chair. Keep a ninety-degree angle between the thighs and spine, still imagining a silver thread lifting you upward. Also keep an L shape between your back and your thighs. This should minimize the chance of any back strain or pain.

Easy Breathing Activities

Here are three breathing activities you can easily engage in throughout the day. Practice them regularly; you'll quickly notice significant, positive results.

Breathing with the Diaphragm

In previous chapters you learned that the two major sources of Qi are the food we eat and the air we breathe. Proper breathing for Qi is abdominal—from the diaphragm. When we breathe with our chest, we use the muscles of our rib cage instead of our diaphragm, the muscle separating the chest from the abdomen. When we breathe from our abdomen, we expand our diaphragm as well as the other abdominal or belly muscles.

Why is this important? According to Chinese medicine—and in keeping with the body's physical layout—the abdomen is the center of the body, the exact, central point being the Dantian point mentioned above. The Qi of all Five Elements is stored in the abdomen, which makes it a microcosm of the body as a whole.

Abdominal breathing does not contradict the scientific model of breathing with the lungs. In fact, it actually increases airflow to the lungs. When we breathe by expanding the chest, the air pressure inside the lungs decreases, creating a vacuum that draws outside air into them. When we breathe more deeply through the diaphragm, we expand our lungs even more, creating an even bigger vacuum and more airflow. In addition, we bring Qi immediately to the center of the body, harmonizing the Qi of all Five Elements.

Qi intake also benefits from your maintaining a good breathing posture, as described above. Major Qi channels pass through the neck and shoulder regions and have various points near the

107

inner angle of the eye, throughout the head, across the back (connecting to all the internal organs), and down the legs. These channels can be constricted by tensing the shoulders. The result of such a Qi disturbance can be anything from a tension headache to an upset stomach.

When we breathe with the diaphragm, it is much more difficult to pull on our shoulders at the same time, so we naturally tend to relax and our whole body stays healthier. At first you will need to tune into your breathing every now and then to make sure you're breathing from the abdomen. After some practice, it becomes second nature. As it does, begin noticing any positive changes in your energy level or physical well-being.

You can make your breathing even more powerful by doing the following: when you breathe in, touch the tip of your tongue on the point where the upper palate (roof of the mouth) meets the upper front teeth. This forms a connection between the Governing Vessel (the major Yang channel, located in the middle of the back) and the Conception Vessel (the major Yin channel, located in the middle of the body's front). As you breathe in, you bring in fresh Qi to balance the Yin and Yang of the whole body.

When you breathe out, open your mouth slightly, gently dropping the tip of your tongue. Let the air out slowly in a stream so fine that it wouldn't disturb a down feather at close range.

Continue taking deep breaths, bringing air in as deeply as possible and letting it out as slowly as possible *without forcing anything*. With practice, you should be able to breathe in and out this way at a rate of four to six smooth breaths per minute.

For optimum health maintenance, you can supplement regular diaphramatic breathing with periodic deep breathing exercises. Here are a couple of simple ones:

The 1:10:4 deep-breathing exercise (the numbers refer to a three-part ratio) is used by many Qigong practitioners. Take a deep breath through your nose into your abdomen, silently counting "1." Hold the breath in your abdomen for as long as possible, up to a count of "10" (ten times longer than the inspiration—guard against speeding up the count!). Then slowly breathe out through your mouth to a count of "4." Again, don't force the effort. You may not initially be able to hold the breath up to 10, or prolong the breathing out up to 4, but that ability will develop with time.

You can combine this exercise with the above-mentioned technique of touching the tip of your tongue to the roof of your mouth during inspiration. Whenever possible during the first few days or weeks of doing this exercise, sit comfortably with good posture in a quiet area so you can concentrate on increasing the amount of time you hold Qi in the abdomen. If you ever feel light-headed or dizzy, you know you are forcing yourself, so go back to a lower ratio (e.g., 1:4:2 instead of 1:6:3) and progress upward more slowly and naturally.

After you become familiar and comfortable with this form of breathing, you will find that you can incorporate it with regular diaphragmatic breathing anytime during the day to increase your Qi. When I move between examining rooms, which takes less than a minute, I routinely massage my hands and do a couple cycles of deep-breathing exercises to recharge my energy battery. This helps me to maintain strong Qi throughout a day of seeing patients.

You can do the same thing as you pause between phone calls, as you walk to meetings, as you sit in traffic—anytime you have a moment and need a boost. If you take a five-minute block of time to do deep breathing continuously, you'll find it peps you up much better than by drinking caffeinated coffee, tea, or soda, or by splashing water on your face!

Microcosmic Breathing

Another form of breathing frequently practiced by Qigong practitioners is what Dr. Chow calls microcosmic breathing. In the last activity, I referred to the Governing Vessel (back body midline) and the Conception Vessel (front body midline) being respectively the major Yang and Yin channels. When Qi flows well in these two master channels, the body's Yin and Yang become balanced. This activity also helps to do just that.

1. Sit in a lotus position on the floor (cross-legged, with each foot resting on the opposite thigh). If you can't assume this position, sit in a chair one-third of the distance back from the edge, maintaining good posture with the spine straight and the feet planted firmly on the floor. Place your hands on your knees with your palms up and your fingers slightly curled.
2. As you breathe in, imagine that the Qi circulates down the Conception Vessel, into the Dantian point (located two inches below the navel and two inches inward), around the genitals to the back, and up the Governing Vessel to the head.
3. As you breathe out, imagine that the Qi moves in the same circuit, so there is no interruption in the microcosmic orbit.
4. Repeat the cycle at least several times per exercise, up to (ideally) five minutes. Remember to keep your spine straight. When you're finished, notice how much more peaceful and energized you feel.

Gentle Cleansing and Qi Strengthening Movements

Here are two easy activities for cleansing the body of toxins and bad Qi and tonifying it with fresh Qi.

Master Zhu's Method

Dr. H. Zhu, the famous Qigong master of Yellow Mountain in China, taught me these simple movements, outlined below, when he was eighty-seven years young. He said, "If you do these movements nine times in the morning and nine times at night, no evil can stay for very long."

The "evil" to which he referred can be anything that can have adverse effects on our health—for example, stress, pollutants or infectious agents from the environment, or an excess of emotions such as anger or frustration. It is important to do what we can to help rid ourselves of this kind of unneeded baggage before it builds up and poses a serious threat. Here's Master Zhu's technique:

1. It's best to do this exercise first thing in the morning. It also can be very effective doing it just before you retire for the night. Ideally you should do this in front of an open window, even if the window is only slightly open; this exposure to fresh air not only "lets out" the evil and helps prevent you from taking it back in, but also restores your Qi connection with the outside world. If it's cold, put on something warm and loose enough to allow for comfortable movement.

2. To cleanse yourself:
   - Stand with your legs shoulder length apart.
   - Bend down and place your palms about one to two inches away from the inside of your lower legs (i.e., your hands should not touch your legs). Move your palms upward along the inside of the legs.
   - Continue moving your palms upward along the sides of the abdomen, the chest, up to the sides of your face, then up around your head to your neck, above the top of the shoulders.
   - As you move your hands down your neck, start turning them outward so that the palms face the front. Using a quick brush stroke motion, quickly "shoosh" evil away to the space in front of you out the window. Make some "shooshing" sound as you do (Master Zhu recommends the Chinese sound "tshuu," meaning "away"). Do this nine

times (9 is considered a heavenly number with magical qualities).

3. Stop for a minute or so to make sure the evils get out.

4. To bring in good (or heavenly) Qi:

  • As you breathe in deeply, raise your arms (palm side up) from each side without bending them until you reach shoulder level. At the same time, slowly raise your heels so that you stand on the balls of your feet. (This massages the KI 1 point.)

  • Continue moving your arms to circle above your head. Pat the space above the crown of your head three times. Do not actually touch your head; just use a gentle patting motion, as if you are pushing Qi into it from Heaven.

  • As you slowly breathe out, gently bring your arms back down to your side, reversing the motion they made before. At the same time, slowly lower your heels to the floor.

  • Do this nine times.

Water Cleansing Qi Exercise

I learned this exercise from Qigong master Adrian Florea when he came to the United States from Romania for the World Congress on Qigong. This exercise is especially helpful for those of you who have difficulty visualizing Qi because it gives you a concrete water image for cleansing yourself.

1. Put your hands together just below your navel, palms up and curved, as if they were forming a cup to hold water.

2. Moving your hands and your elbows so that your two forearms maintain a reasonably straight line, come up the midline of your body, along the Conception Vessel line, until the "cup" reaches the mouth.

3. Opening your mouth, imagine you are drinking Qi (or water) from your hands for three to five seconds.

4. As you slowly breathe out through your mouth, slowly turn your palms downward and reverse the movement you made in motion 2 above.

As you do this, imagine that the Qi (or water) you drank is cleansing your body and washing away everything you don't need down your legs and through the balls of your feet into the Earth.

Repeat the exercises three to nine times.

Meditations

From the standpoint of Chinese medicine, meditation is another invaluable component of maintaining health through balancing the Qi flow. There are many meditation methods and styles—including Taoist, Yogic, Hindu, Buddhist, and Qigong—that help reinforce Qi and get rid of unhealthy physical, mental, and emotional symptoms. Many specific meditations can be found in books, periodicals, and tapes at bookstores, libraries, and health-related or spiritual centers. You may want to experiment with different styles, methods, or meditations on your own to determine what best suits you. Meanwhile, here are some basic, widely used meditations to get you started.

Simple Meditation

In this exercise, you use your deep breathing to go into meditation.

Choose a quiet place where you will not be disturbed by telephones or outside noises. Sit in a lotus or half-lotus position, or sit comfortably in a chair, keeping your spine straight. Put your hands on your knees, palms up. Close your eyes. Now choose one of the breathing exercises, exaggerate it, and just concentrate on your breathing. For example, if you choose the microcosmic breathing, try to gradually make the cycle bigger, much bigger than your actual body size. Forget your exact physical form for the time being. Be patient. Don't be discouraged if you cannot do it right away. After you do it several times, you will notice that the cycle takes longer to complete because you have grown so much taller. See if you can fill up the room or fill up the house. The sky's the limit!

Soon you will be in a state where noises or distractions do not bother you. You don't notice them because you are too big for them. This image will be translated metaphorically in your life, when you are too big to be stressed by the small stuff that bogs down others. You can find peace between Heaven and Earth.

Give yourself a big smile as you come out of this meditation.

The Chow Five-Element Meditation

This meditation, a condensed version of the full one developed by Dr. Chow and appearing in *Miracle Healing from China—Qigong*, takes about twenty minutes if you do all three stages. If you have less time, you can do just Stage One or Stages One and Two.

Stage One:
1. *On the floor, using a cushion under the buttocks if desired, sit in a lotus position or a half-lotus position (only one foot needs to rest on the opposite thigh; the other can rest on the floor). If you can't, sit in any cross-legged position. You can also sit in a chair, as described above in the last breathing activity.*
2. *Keep your head facing straight forward. Visualize being pulled upward by a silver thread coming up from the center of the Earth, passing through your tailbone, up your spine, through*

the DU 20 point at the top of your head, and on up into the sky.

Now visualize a second silver thread coming from your Dantian point and pulling you forward, slightly tilting your pelvis so the torso of your body sits on it properly.

Finally, drop a silver thread from the shoulders downward in back of you to keep your shoulders comfortably back and down.

3. *Now breathe deeply and easily with your diaphragm, concentrating on the in-and-out movement and on comfortably maximizing your lung capacity.*

During inspiration, breathe in through the nose while lightly touching the tip of your tongue to the roof of your mouth where it meets the upper front teeth.

During expiration, open your mouth slightly, drop your tongue, and breathe out through your mouth, relaxing your jaw muscles and allowing your whole body to hang loosely from that first, main silver thread.

As you breathe, feel the Qi circulating continuously down your Governing Vessel in front, through your Dantian, around your genitals, and up your Conception Vessel in back, and so on, in a never-ending cycle. Then feel the vibrant Qi coursing through every muscle, tendon, bone, and cell in your body.

4. *As you continue breathing, acknowledge each thought that flows through your mind and let it go. Also acknowledge any noise and let it fall into the background.*

Let yourself experience whatever you are feeling, whether it's physical, emotional, or spiritual, pleasant or unpleasant. Don't avoid it, deny it, or crowd it out. Feel what it truly is, then let it go. Eventually you will feel warmth flowing through your body, relaxing tense muscles.

If you experience movement, let yourself flow with it while remaining in the same basic posture. You are responding to the swaying of the atmospheric Qi around you. If you experience sound, don't hinder expressing it, as long as that expression is natural and doesn't break the meditative state.

Stage Two:
Having centered and maximized your Qi, call upon the universal Qi by getting in touch with each of the Five Elements: Water, Wood, Earth, Metal, and Fire. Think about each of these elements, in order, for one minute, letting yourself sense all the images associated with it that easily come to mind before moving on to the next element.

As you think about each element, call upon its power to reinforce your own Qi to heal yourself. When you have finished, let yourself feel how good it feels to connect with the universal Qi, and let yourself feel the power of all the elements you've visualized.

Stage Three:
1. *To help cleanse yourself of any internal problem—physical, mental, emotional, or spiritual—first visualize it as something concrete and unpleasant (e.g., an angry dog, a gray cloud, or a pile of garbage) existing in any particular place inside your body except your Dantian.*
2. *As you breathe and hold this image in your mind, move healthy, vibrant Qi from your Dantian to that place. Once the Qi is there, imagine it shoving the unpleasant image directly out of your body, by the shortest route possible.*
3. *Now visualize a concrete image of the health coming into your body (e.g., glowing lights or beautiful flowers). As you breathe, spread this image throughout your body, mind, and spirit until you become that image.*

   If you want, repeat the process with another problem that's bothering you. Don't worry if you have unpleasant feelings during this stage of the meditation, or if you temporarily get distracted or fall asleep. Whatever you experience is what you need at the time.

When you are ready to come out of the Five-Elements meditation, or any stage of it, or any other meditation, first concentrate on taking a few deeper diaphragmatic breaths and enjoy the sense of harmony within yourself. Then encircle the universal Qi in one complete breath by bringing your arms out to each side, encircling them up and forward, and bringing them down, right hand on top of the left for men and left hand on top of the right for women, toward the Dantian. Do this three times, then relax with your palms turned upward in your lap. Slowly open your eyes, and enjoy the harmony of being in tune with yourself and the universe.

The White Light Meditation

Imagine a white light (positive Qi) entering your body through the DU 20 point on your head. The light slowly starts filling you with warmth, permeating different parts of your body. As it does, it pushes all darkness (negative Qi) out. In time, your whole body is filled with the light, and nothing negative can enter it. Stay with this feeling for as long as you want.

The Magnetic Cord Meditation

Imagine a silver thread extending from the center of the Earth, coming up through your tailbone and spine, through the DU point in your head, and on into the sky. Imagine it is a magnetic cord that can absorb everything toxic inside you: whatever you do not want, such as physical or emotional pain; whatever you are ready to release, such as grief; and whatever no longer serves you, such as anger. Let the cord absorb all these things and then ground them into the center of the Earth, never to return, while

117

simultaneously pulling down golden sunlight from Heaven to fill up your body.

Movement Activities

The Chinese arts of Qigong and Tai Chi are movement practices that enhance body flexibility and control, maintain health, and relieve stress. Both practices have many schools, each with a different style and group of exercises. I'll give you a few simple examples from Dr. Chow to get you started. If you are interested, you can look into Qigong and Tai Chi classes where you live, and pursue more.

The best time to do these exercises is early in the morning, to get your Qi energy working after a long period of rest. However, doing them at any time of day is beneficial. As with all forms of exercise, consistency and persistence are the keys to results.

The Arc Stance

1. Stand with your feet a shoulder distance apart.
2. As you begin breathing in, slowly bring your arms up, holding each arm straight out to the side with the palm turned upward.
3. Continue moving your arms upward until they come above your head and the palms meet. At the same time, raise your heels until you're standing on your toes.
4. As you begin slowly breathing out through your mouth, move your arms back down with your palms turned downward, reversing the arc. As they descend, slowly lower your heels until your feet are firmly back on the ground.

Do the Arc Stance at least three times a day. Ten would be ideal.

The Horse Stance

The Horse Stance is an exercise to develop stamina and to increase Qi to the Dantian.

1. Begin by standing with your feet together. Place your weight on your heels and rotate your toes outward until they form a line as straight across as possible.
2. Put your weight on your toes, and rotate your heels out so your toes are pointed slightly in. You should end up standing with your feet about as far apart as your shoulders and slightly pigeon-toed.
3. Activate your Qi through the Lao Gong point (see the section "Soothing Massages" later in this chapter). Then hold your arms out at heart level, with your fingers pointing toward each other about one foot apart, palms facing your torso. Drop your shoulders back and relax your muscles.
4. Bend your knees slightly while keeping your spine straight. Breathe slowly and rhythmically with the diaphragm. Concentrate on your breathing, and focus on the Qi at the Dantian point.
5. Maintain the posture for as long as you can tolerate. Gradually lengthen the time as you become stronger.

This posture may seem awkward at first, but you will notice Qi moving up to the face and head and throughout the body. You may even become temporarily flushed, sweaty, and red-faced. Be patient with this stance—it is excellent for cardiovascular circulation.

The Infinity Stance

1. Get into the Horse Stance (see above, steps 1 to 4).
2. Keeping the spine straight and the pelvis loose, put your hands on your sacrum, over the Bladder channel.

119

3. Make an infinity (or sideways figure eight) pattern with your pelvis: move the pelvis forward, then right, then back, then left, then forward, then left, then back, then right, then forward, and so on. Do this in multiples of three, depending on your time (up to infinity!). Be sure that your pelvis is loose and relaxed and that the infinity pattern is big. There should be at least nine inches between the pelvis in the front position and in the back position.

The "Connect with Heaven and Earth" Stance

1. In a standing position, with your feet a shoulder length apart and your arms at your side, turn your palms upward and pointing straight out to the side.
2. As you inhale, slowly raise your arms out to the side, drawing a large circle, until they are above the back of your head with the palms together.

    At the same time, imagine you are sweeping pure energy from Heaven—Heavenly Qi—to the DU 20 point at the crown of your head.
3. As you finish inhaling, bring your palm-to-palm hands slowly down in front of you until they are opposite your mouth. Then turn your palms toward your face and begin slowly exhaling through your mouth. Continue exhaling as you move your hands (now separating) and arms down to your side.

    At the same time, imagine that Heavenly Qi is moving down your body, calming you physically, mentally, emotionally, and spiritually and washing away toxic energy through your feet into the Earth.
4. Restart by bringing your palms out and breathing in. Do the stance in multiples of three, depending on how much time you have. As you become more familiar with it, the arm motion will become more continuous and fluid.

Soothing Massages

Our hands are more than mechanical structures that enable us to pick up, punch, or hold things. We express with our hands. We heal with our hands. We make human connections with our hands. As I mentioned in chapter 1, our hands also are microsystems that map out our entire body and its energy systems. Massaging by hand is therefore a very powerful, stimulating, and reintegrating activity. It can effectively treat any area of discomfort that we can reach on ourselves or on someone else. The shoulders and the back of the neck, for example, are common areas of tension and distress. We can massage them by kneading them or simply by placing our warm (i.e., Qi-activated) hands over the area of tightness or pain.

First I'll show you how to activate Qi in the hands via the Lao Gong point. Many Qigong masters, including Dr. Chow, advocate this. Then I'll describe good, basic massages for the abdomen, back, and Qi channels.

Activating Qi in the Hands

1. Start by just rubbing your hands together, and then gently kneading each palm and back of the hand in turn.
2. Using either one of your hands, make a fist with your fingers. The point in the palm of the hand between the middle and the fourth (ring) finger is the Lao Gong point, translated as "Hardworking" point. It corresponds to the middle of the abdomen on the hand microsystem.
3. Line up the Lao Gong points on your palms, then rub your palms together vigorously so the Lao Gong points on each palm touch as you do so. The warmth you feel—on the first try or after practicing for a while—is Qi.

4. After you've activated Qi, test for it by holding your palms facing toward each other about one or two inches apart. Focus on the sensation between the palms. Do you feel heat or tingling, pulsating sensations? If so, you know you've activated Qi. There may even be similar physical sensations elsewhere in the body.

Don't worry if you don't feel Qi right away. Keep practicing and you will eventually sense it.

Now I'm going to give you two simple massages that will help you maintain your own health and the health of your loved ones. Although it's important to have good, strong Qi in your hands for these massages, it's equally critical to put your mind into a healing mode, because our minds and bodies are so intimately linked. Think positive, healing thoughts such as "This massage will help me [or someone else] feel better." Don't massage yourself or others if you are angry, stressed, or very tired. Instead, take a few moments to calm and strengthen yourself with rest or meditation.

Abdominal Massage

Abdominal Qi needs to flow smoothly because the abdomen is where food is digested and where all Five Elements of Qi concentrate. After activating the Qi in your hands, massage the area around the navel with either your palm or your four fingertips bunched together. Make thirty to fifty clockwise motions and then the same number of counterclockwise motions.

This technique works for general maintenance and for most common abdominal problems. However, in cases of diarrhea, only massage counterclockwise; in cases of constipation, only clockwise. If the abdominal area is too painful to massage, you can simply put your activated hand over the area of pain or brush over it lightly (whichever feels better).

Back Massage (cannot be self-administered)

The Bladder meridian on the back has points called Back Shu points that connect with all the organs in the body (see the diagram in appendix D). In addition, there are four sets of points along these channels that have been found to improve immunity. Qi flows in these channels from the head toward the legs.

To administer a healing back massage that stimulates all these points, use your palm or four fingers together to massage firmly downward alongside the spine from the shoulder to the hip region (the Bladder meridian). Then lift your hands and, starting at the shoulder, massage down again.

Do not move your hands back up the spine, because you would thereby be moving Qi in the wrong direction. Also avoid massaging the spine itself when you come down, because the Qi in the Governing Vessel, which runs along the spine, flows from the sacrum upward to the head.

Do this massage thirty to fifty times once or twice a day. The person you massage will feel more energy and less stress and will get sick less often. If possible, get him or her to do it for you so you know personally what I'm talking about!

Healing Sound Activities

Sounds affect us physically and emotionally every day. Think of how you respond to the sound of car horns honking, the scratching of fingernails across a blackboard, birds chirping in the morning, rock music, a soft flute, a jackhammer. So what role does sound play in Chinese medicine?

Qi is energy, and energy is a wave. Sound is also a wave. Chinese medicine maintains that certain sound wave vibrations can heal organs on the cellular level. That's because the Qi of each organ's cells generates a specific wavelength. A sound we make that resonates with that wavelength can therefore tonify (or strengthen) it. Western science offers its own explanation: two wavelengths superimposed on each other increase the magnitude of the wave.

According to Chinese medicine, when Qi is weak in an organ's cells, the wavelength amplitude is lower, so the healing process is assisted by reinforcing that amplitude vocally. Even a whisper can help.

The five prolonged sounds listed below are for tonifying the Yin organs, which are the more important ones. The stronger the cells are in these organs, the less likely they are to suffer disease. Because Yin organ Qi is also associated with emotions, sound therapy can help keep a person emotionally as well as physically well balanced. Intone each of these sounds for several ten-to-twenty-second rounds, several times a day, and you'll keep yourself humming!

1. *AHHHHHH—Heart:* Put you hand on your heart and say AHHHHHH loudly. Feel the vibration, so you have a tactile sense of what it's like. Heart energy is connected with the circulatory system and the Mind as a whole, in particular the emotion of joy. Can you think of a time when you saw something you liked and said "Ahhhhhh!"? Right then and there, you opened up your heart for joy.

2. *SHEEEEEE—Lungs:* Place your hand on your chest and feel the vibration as you loudly say SHEEEIII. You can feel the difference between this sound and AHHHHHH. It vibrates deeper in the chest and is good for any lung-related problem such as coughing, wheezing, congestion, and so on. It's also beneficial for people who need to let go of their grief or sadness.

3. *WUUUUUUU—Digestive System:* Place your hand on your abdomen and feel the vibration as you loudly say WUUUU-UUU, taking care to keep your voice low-pitched. Sense how deep this sound feels. It is as if you can feel it going all the

way down into the Earth. This sound benefits abdominal problems such as stomachache or diarrhea. It also helps resolve obsessiveness and stressed-out feelings.

4. *JIAAAAAOOOOO (pronounced GEE-A [as in hay]- OOO [as in moo]-OH [short-oh sound])—Liver:* This is a relatively difficult vibration to feel, just as many Liver conditions are difficult to sense or diagnose. In addition to strengthening the Liver in general, it also helps treat anger or irritability. Many people use the sound during their Qigong or Tai Chi exercises.

5. *FOOOOOOO (as in moo; does not end in short-oh sound)—Kidney:* This sound vibrates deep in the lower back. In addition to helping Kidney-related physical and emotional problems (such as fear), it strengthens development in children and sexual energy in adults. It also helps slow down the post-forty aging process.

Because the Kidney is such an important organ, it's worth spending extra time and care to make sure the sound works its best. Find a quiet place and sit comfortably cross-legged or on the edge of a chair. Warm your hands and place them on your lower back above your hipbone. Then focus on your concern: your physical problem (e.g., nephritis or an infection); something you fear or need encouragement to face; or your desire to increase your sexual energy or slow down the aging process. Then repeat the FOOOOOOO sound several times. Even if you can't go through this process, however, it still helps simply to intone the sound, even if it's merely a whisper.

Final Touches for Good Health

Chinese medicine looks at our being as a physical, mental, emotional, and spiritual whole. Just as negative thoughts and feelings can be injurious to our health, so positive ones can bring us into a healthier balance. Low self-esteem is a major affliction for people of all ages, and it's at the root of many crippling, whole-person illnesses, including eating disorders and alcoholism. Just focusing on even the smallest positive images about ourselves and our situation can boost our Qi, and this includes saying to ourselves things like "I can do it," "I will feel stronger," "I am going to help myself."

On a more physical level, it helps a lot to give and receive hugs. Dr. Chow recommends at least eight heart-to-heart body hugs a day! They not only bring the huggers closer together, but also literally increase each hugger's Qi energy, improving such vital signs as heart rate and blood pressure. Recent scientific studies have established that hugging even has a positive effect on white blood cells, the body's front-line infection fighters, and on the level of endorphins, the body's natural pain-relievers. A far greater blessing, however, may be the increased sense of being loved and valued that each hugger receives.

In addition, both Chinese and Western medicine recognize the value of smiles and laughter in healing and in maintaining good health. At the end of a meditation or exercise session, for example, give yourself a big smile as a reward. It's also wise to be playful each day, and to make sure your reading and viewing diet includes a healthy dose of humorous material.

You are now equipped with all sorts of quick and easy things you can do almost anywhere and at any time to keep yourself and others healthy. You may forget to carry pills and potions, but your hands, body, and voice are always available. Hopefully, now that you know how much day-to-day mindfulness helps in Chinese health care, you also always have your wits about you!

PART II

The Integrative Chinese and Western Treatment Guide

CHAPTER 6

Healing Common
Health Problems

By regularly combining Western and Chinese treatments to cope with illnesses or injuries, you'll benefit from safer, quicker, more comprehensive healings; you'll also gain a much deeper long-term understanding of how to maintain a healthy lifestyle. To this end, this chapter offers a guide for treating more than fifty common health problems using simple Western and Chinese practices.

The Importance of Acupressure

Throughout the entries in this guide, the Chinese practice I most frequently advise is acupressure, a massage administered by the fingers or the hand to particular points or areas on the body in accordance with the specific health problem. Here are guidelines for massaging these points or areas as effectively as possible:

1. *Warm your hands before massaging.* To increase the Qi in your hands, warm them by rubbing them together. For maximum benefits, warm your Lao Gong point as described in chapter 4.

2. *Put yourself in a positive mental state for massage.* Remember that since your mind and body are connected, what you think or feel will influence your massage. Take a moment to ensure that you are calm, focused, and have loving intentions for healing yourself (if self-massaging) or the other person.

3. *Massage the skin directly for best results.* Massage is more effective when you actually make physical contact with the skin. The warmth of your hands and the feeling of touch enhance the healing as well as the enjoyment of massage. In instances when you cannot remove clothing, massaging through clothing still can be beneficial, since your electromagnetic field extends beyond the physical boundaries of skin and clothing.

4. *Do not apply lotions for massage.* You do not need to apply lotions, creams, oils, or ointments to the massage area. However, if your hands are dry, or if you prefer the feel of oil or lotion, you can use organic ones and avoid applying chemicals, which may interfere with natural Qi contact.

5. *Assume the most comfortable or convenient position for the massage.* Use your own best judgment about the situation. If you're massaging someone's back, it's best for the person to be lying down. If the person is sitting in a chair, it's preferable for him or her to lean forward on something like a pillow on a table so that he or she can safely fall asleep. When you massage someone's abdomen, the person should be lying down in bed or leaning back in a comfortable chair. Massaging the legs, arms, hands, or head can be done in whatever position works well.

6. *Take advantage of any convenient time and place for massage.*

The recommended daily massage or massages for a particular health problem can be beneficial at any time during the day, and you can administer them as often as you wish in any given day. You cannot overdose on massage—the more you do, the more benefit there is. If you are massaging to prevent pain, for example, do it whenever you have time!

Purists massage according to the hourly schedule of maximum-minimum activity for a particular organ system, as discussed in chapter 1. For example, the Stomach has maximum activity between 7:00 A.M. and 9:00 A.M., so this time period is best for massages relating to Stomach problems. However, following such a schedule can be difficult.

As a general rule, massaging to treat a particular illness tends to be especially effective when the symptoms of that illness are active. Other kinds of massage can be timed logically to suit their purpose. For example, if you have insomnia, you will want to do the self-massage that helps you sleep *just before* bedtime. It's usually better to massage between or before meals rather than during or right after them, because you don't want the massage stimulation to interfere with Digestive Qi.

The optimum length of time to massage in a single session can vary according to the circumstances. Acute symptoms such as headaches or abdominal pain may require twenty or more minutes of massage—about the time it takes a medicated analgesic tablet to take effect. The younger the person is, the less time it can take for massage to be effective. Children generally require only half as much time as adults, and infants often need just a few seconds per point.

When you do acupressure regularly to balance chronic disorders, one to three minutes per point usually is advisable, depending on the number of points you need to massage and the amount of time you have. It's better to do what you can than to do nothing at all. Massaging for a shorter time more frequently—such as a minute per point, three times a day—can be very effective.

A major blessing of acupressure is that you can massage yourself whenever and wherever you want. For example, you can massage your hands, wrists, and arms while you are waiting in the car for a red light to change. You also can discreetly massage your hands while attending meetings, riding in an elevator, or even talking with people. One of my patients with chronic headaches regularly presses the LI 4 point on his hand during elevator rides to and from his fourteenth-floor office. To anyone else in the elevator, he just looks as if he is holding his briefcase with both hands.

7. *Be sure to massage in the recommended direction.* I provide specific instructions about the direction to massage in each relevant guide entry. As a general rule, massaging in a clockwise direction (i.e., with the massaged person as the "clock") tonifies or strengthens a point or area by putting Qi into it. Massaging in a counterclockwise direction takes Qi out of the point or area, which is appropriate in cases of Qi stagnation.

8. *Use the massage technique that's appropriate: for spots, for areas of the body, or for the hand.*

   * *Massaging acupressure spots.* Apply firm pressure with the thumb, index, and middle fingers bunched together or, alternatively, with the first knuckle (*above* the back side of the hand) of the index or middle finger. The pressure should be firm to the point of feeling soreness but not pain. Soreness is to be expected because the relevant points usually are made tender by the existing health problems, but massaging the points should soon bring comfort. You can just press on the point and keep pressure on it, or you can move your finger or fingers or knuckle back and forth to stimulate it, or you can rotate your finger or fingers in a clockwise or counterclockwise motion, as directed.

   * *Massaging areas of the body.* Treatment guide entries often

suggest massaging an entire area of the body, such as the upper back or abdomen. You can massage these areas with the palm of your hand, with four fingers bunched together, or (for large areas) with both the palms and the fingers, applying firm pressure as you do. Just be sure to follow the recommended direction.

- *Massaging micromeridians on the hand.* These lines require only gentle strokes, because the microsystem points are much smaller and closer to the surface. Usually you can massage an entire micromeridian with just the index finger. Again, be sure to follow the recommended direction. As a general rule, you stroke in the direction of Qi flow to tonify the micromeridian, and against it to sedate the flow.

9. *Four general massages for overall maintenance of health.* Chinese medicine and Western medicine both emphasize the importance of health maintenance and preventive medicine. In keeping with these emphases, here are four general massages that can keep you healthy and fit and prevent problems.

A. *Massaging the master points for the Three Burners.* Chapter 2 notes that detecting temperature differences on the Three Burners can help assess where problems exist. For example, coldness in the Middle Burner may indicate simultaneous digestive problems even though there are Lung (Upper Burner) symptoms. The Three Burners have divisions on the front of the body in keeping with the diagram.

Each Burner has a "master point" that influences the entire Burner. Massaging these three master points routinely can help maintain overall harmony in the Three Burners and their corresponding organs.
- CV 17: Upper Burner
- CV 12: Middle Burner
- CV 6: Lower Burner

133

THREE BURNER DIAGRAM

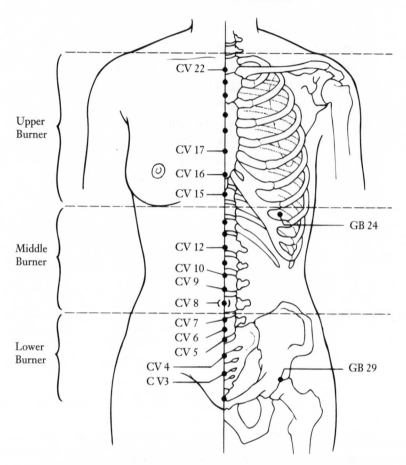

B. *Massaging the "Back Shu" points for all the organs.* The back has two Bladder lines: the inner Bladder has "shu" or "transport" points that transport Qi to all the organs; the outer Bladder line has points with spiritual values.

The Bladder channel flows from top to bottom, from the shoulders to the hips. By massaging these channels regularly in the direction of flow (i.e., in the downward direction), you can help your loved one maintain harmonious

BLADDER "SHU" POINTS

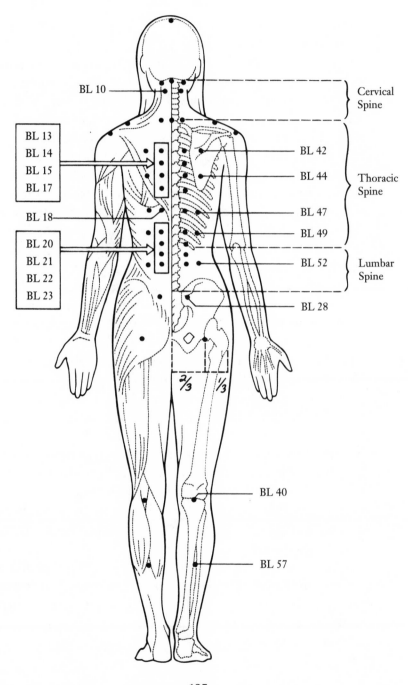

BL 10

BL 13
BL 14
BL 15
BL 17

BL 18

BL 20
BL 21
BL 22
BL 23

Cervical
Spine

BL 42

BL 44

Thoracic
Spine

BL 47

BL 49

BL 52

Lumbar
Spine

BL 28

⅔   ⅓

BL 40

BL 57

Qi flow to all the organs and achieve spiritual balance, the firm basis for good health.

First, warm your hands. Then, using either your palms or your four fingers together, apply firm pressure and massage next to the spine from the shoulder toward the hip. Lift your hands, start at the shoulder, and come down again. Do not massage backward, from the hip to the shoulder; otherwise you will reverse Qi flow. Also, avoid massaging the spine downward, since Qi in the Governing Vessels in the midline of the back flows from bottom to top. This massage is especially effective for general health maintenance in children. Do fifty strokes once or twice a day, whichever your schedule allows. The massage usually takes two to three minutes per session.

Since you cannot massage your own back, you can use the hand microsystem and massage the back of your hands from the web spaces around the middle finger toward the wrist, next to the spine. On the hand, the spine corresponds to the middle of the back of the hand from the wrist to the tip of the third finger.

C. *Massaging the abdomen.* Since the abdomen is a microsystem that contains Qi from all Five Elements, massaging the abdomen regularly can also ensure overall smooth and harmonious Qi flow. This massage is also discussed for abdominal pain and for a variety of digestive problems, which often are at the root of many disorders that affect even nondigestive organs. According to Chinese medicine, a healthy digestive system helps promote good overall health and fitness.

First, warm your hands by rubbing them together to activate the Lao Gong point. Then slowly and gently massage the abdominal area using circular, clockwise motions (think of the left side as three o'clock). Massage in this direction twenty-five times. Then massage counterclockwise, in the reverse direction, twenty-five times. Avoid direct contact with the navel (the "belly button"), which may cause discomfort. Move your hands as far up as the tip of the sternum, as far to each side as a line drawn from the armpit down the sides of the body, and as low as the pubic area. Massage once or twice a day. Remember, this is only for health maintenance in the absence of abdominal or digestive symptoms. If you have symptoms, follow the suggestions in the guide for specific massages.

D. *Massaging the Five-Element master points.* In chapter 2 I described the Five-Element relationship of the organ system. In addition, acupressure/acupuncture points also have Five-Element designations such as Water-Liver, Wood-Liver, and Earth-Liver points, for all the Qi channels, and they are all located on the extremities between the elbows and the fingers, and the knees and the toes. Massaging the segments of the channels regularly can prevent Qi flow problems. You can do this form of massage on yourself or on a loved one.

Massaging leg master points. Warm your hands first. With one hand, massage the inside of the leg from the toes to the knees in an upward direction, and massage the outside of the leg from the knee to the toes in a downward direction. You can do this simultaneously on yourself and on someone else. The outside of the leg has three Yang channels: Stomach, Gallbladder, and Bladder. The inside of the leg has three Yin channels: Liver, Spleen, and Kidney.

Massaging arm master points. You can massage both sides on someone else and only one side at a time on yourself. Massage the inside of the arm from the elbow downward toward the fingertips, and massage the outside of the arm from the fingertips to the elbow. The outside of the arm has three Yang channels: Large Intestine, Small

Intestine, and Triple Burner. The inside of the arm has three Yin channels: Lung, Heart, and Master of the Heart (Pericardium). Do each side twenty-five to fifty strokes once or twice a day. This process should take only a few minutes at a time.

These are four massages for general balance. You do not need to do all four massages every day. Usually one or two massages a day is sufficient. You can also alternate: one day do the back massage, another day do the Five-Element massage. Ask your loved one to do them on you—enjoy the feel of loving touches that will help keep you healthy as well.

10. *Acupressure points*.

For a full discussion of acupressure points, see appendix D.

Abdominal Pain

Symptoms

General or localized pain below the chest cavity and above the groin, including the stomach and intestines, urinary and reproductive systems. The pain can be sharp or dull and may be accompanied by nausea, vomiting, diarrhea, or fever.

Description

Abdominal pain can be divided into two categories: (1) acute, recent, or sudden-onset pain and (2) recurrent, chronic pain.

Acute, recent, or sudden-onset pain. The pain comes on quickly, maybe generalized or transient (moving around), and is sometimes accompanied by belching (excessive gas), flatulence (excessive gas), vomiting, diarrhea, or fever.

It is important to rule out possible appendicitis, which may begin with generalized pain but usually or eventually becomes localized pain in the lower right abdomen. Severe or sharp pain may also signal gallstones, kidney stones, intestinal obstructions, or ulcers. If you have severe abdominal pain that persists, consult a physician immediately.

In Western medicine, acute abdominal pain is commonly attributed to a harmful infectious agent, such as a virus, parasite, or bacteria that causes inflammation, to food poisoning from bacterial toxins, or to stress or drugs. Other common causes include constipation and menstrual cramps. Chinese medicine offers a broader perspective. In addition to, or instead of, the causes just mentioned, two other factors—coldness or dampness—can cause acute abdominal pain by creating a Qi imbalance.

Coldness contracts the energy channels and blood vessels so that less blood and Qi are delivered to the tissues, resulting in pain. The coldness itself can come either from the environment (cold weather or a body chilled by something cold, such as swimming in cold water) or from food (excessive intake of cold foods). For this reason, many people get cold-related abdominal pain in the summertime after swimming and after drinking iced beverages. In addition, menstruation and childbirth predispose women to this kind of pain. Often a cold-related abdominal pain occurs specifically in the upper part of the abdomen (epigastrium) and is accompanied by diarrhea.

In Chinese medicine, the navel—the center of the body—is considered highly susceptible to coldness in the environment. Therefore, to help avoid cold-related abdominal pain, it's wise to protect the navel from direct exposure to cold weather and cooling winds or water. This is especially important for infants and young children, who have more sensitive systems.

Dampness causes abdominal pain by clogging up the energy channels and, as a result, slowing or obstructing Qi flow. Dampness on the ground can penetrate the body through the legs, which are the primary locations of both the Stomach and the Spleen digestive channels. Dampness also enters the body—and, sooner or later, the digestive channels—through the pores of the skin. This means that people are predisposed to damp-related abdominal pain if they live in a damp basement or a humid climate, or if they don't dry themselves quickly and adequately after swimming or getting soaked in the rain. Food intake may be another factor: too many dairy products or phlegm-producing foods can create an internal dampness. A viral or bacterial infection—for example, from food poisoning—causes acute dampness. Abdominal pain related to dampness may be accompanied by a feeling of fullness or heaviness and sometimes by diarrhea.

In addition to infectious agents, coldness, or dampness, improper eating can cause acute abdominal pain. As mentioned above, excessive intake of cold foods can trigger cold-related pain; phlegm-producing foods can cause damp-related pain. However, abdominal discomfort in general can quickly be caused by eating too much or too little food, an unbalanced variety of foods, or an abundance of processed foods.

Two other actions can cause abdominal distress: eating too much, and eating too little. Eating too much overloads the Stomach, which produces a bloated feeling in the upper abdomen, burping, and a sour taste in the mouth. Eating too little—which can include either fasting, eating tiny amounts, or following a diet that is very restrictive (e.g., low-fat, vegetarian, etc.)—can cause not only a nutritional imbalance but also pain in the upper abdomen.

The same applies to a recent diet that's disproportionately geared to only one or two types of food. Consuming too many hot foods (e.g., spices, beef, and alcohol) can result in a burning sensation in the upper abdomen. A somewhat duller pain may be caused by eating too many sweet and greasy foods or too many processed foods (specifically, foods that contain chemical preservatives and artificial food colorings). Besides directly inducing abdominal pain, processed foods can generate allergic reactions, emotional imbalances, and irritation of the stomach lining—all of which can contribute to abdominal discomfort.

An individual's manner of eating may also lead to upper

abdominal pain. Grabbing a hamburger on the go or tackling a rough assignment immediately after a meal doesn't give Digestive Qi enough time or peace to do its proper work. Eating while watching TV decreases Qi for digestion, since Qi that is needed for processing food is diverted to processing the TV program. Dining or snacking late at night stirs up Qi for digestion at precisely the time when the entire body should be preparing for rest—the therapeutic Yin cycle of less activity. An upsetting disturbance of Qi also can occur whenever a person eats at irregular intervals or radically changes diet from one day to the next.

Recurrent, chronic pain: Rather than being acute, recent, or sudden-onset, the abdominal pain may be a dull, achy one that can be localized or generalized, episodic or recurrent. Western diagnosis includes inflammatory bowel disease, ulcers, polyps, parasitic infections, and cancer. Frequently, chronic abdominal pain can result from stress. In this case, laboratory testing often cannot find a physical cause and the pain is diagnosed as psychosomatic.

Chinese medicine attributes this pain to persistent internal coldness, possibly due to repeated (or habitual) improper food ingestion, such as eating excessively large amounts of cold foods, or else eating too fast and thus not allowing enough time for food to be converted to Nutritive Qi. In either case, a general cooling of the digestive area occurs that repeatedly disrupts the flow of Digestive Qi.

This description helps explain why recurrent, chronic abdominal pain may be related to stress. Aside from the fact that stress interferes with the harmonious flow of Qi in general (including Digestive Qi), people under stress tend to ignore good diet practices and skip, rush through, pick at, or overdo meals.

Chinese medicine consistently emphasizes the vital role that emotional balance plays in a person's overall well-being. This emphasis includes his or her abdominal health. Too much experience of any tense emotion—whether it's anger, fear, sadness, or frustration—can lead to chronic pain, often in the upper abdomen and extending to the sides. Sometimes the pain is accompanied by loose stools.

Indeed, balance in every area of life is critical to a well-functioning abdomen. A habit of working too late, exercising too hard, or loafing around too much, combined with poor dietary habits and emotional stress (which are, after all, logical consequences of such behaviors) can easily cause problems in the digestive tract.

To examine either acute or chronic abdominal pain from the perspective of Chinese medicine, use your hand to feel for temperature differences throughout the abdominal area. It's best to use the more sensitive back of your hand when examining others. When examining yourself, you can curl your fingers and use the back of them or you can use your palm, although the latter may give slighter warmer readings. Note any coldness between the lower tip of the sternum (or breastbone, down the center of the rib cage) and the navel. This area is the Middle Burner in Chinese medicine—the area for digestive function. Coldness indicates a lack of Qi, and an uneven distribution of coldness indicates an imbalance in the flow of Qi.

Western Treatment

For either acute or chronic pain: Increase rest and relaxation, reduce stress, and eliminate foods that are acidic, high in caffeine, or difficult to digest. If there's diarrhea, increase intake of fluids to replenish body fluids. Specific treatments are prescribed for particular chronic conditions, such as antacid for ulcers. Be careful when you take over-the-counter medications to reduce pain, gas, and diarrhea, that you are not masking symptoms that can delay proper diagnosis.

Chinese Treatment

For either acute or chronic pain:

Administer a general massage. First, warm your hands by activating the Lao Gong point (see chapter 5). Then slowly and gently massage the abdominal area using circular, clockwise motions (think of the left side as three o'clock). If diarrhea is a symptom, then massage in a counterclockwise direction. Avoid direct contact with the navel, as this may cause discomfort. Move your hands as far up as the tip of the sternum, as far to each side as a line drawn from the armpit down the sides of the body, and as low as the pubic area. Massage fifty strokes once or twice a day.

Massage the following points and body areas, as appropriate for the symptoms:
- CV 12, the Middle Burner, to improve Qi flow
- ST 36, the master immunity point, to strengthen Qi
- SP 6 to help move and transform Digestive Qi
- ST 40 to clear dampness
- P 6 to alleviate nausea and vomiting
- LR 3 to reduce stress and anger
- LI 4 if there is a headache
- CV 6 if there are loose stools
- the hand micromeridian F, which corresponds to the Spleen channel, massage from the tip toward the palm (do not go backward)
- the hand micromeridian E, which corresponds to the Stomach channel; massage from the palm toward the tip (opposite the F channel above)

Also, do the following treatments:
- Keep the abdomen warm, especially the navel.
- Avoid any foods or liquids that are chilled, frozen, or iced. Also avoid raw fruits and vegetables, including salads. Eat foods at room temperature or cooked.
- Choose foods from the warm list.

Consult a physician if symptoms last longer than a week or if the following symptoms occur: persistent fever, more localized pain, sharp pain, or inability to keep down liquids.

Alcohol and Alcoholism

Symptoms

Symptoms vary according to level of drunkenness, which depends on the amount of alcohol consumed and the individual's tolerance. Symptoms range from giddiness, withdrawal, and slurred speech to impairment of judgment, rationalization, and coordination and to passing out from inebriation. Hangover symptoms include headache, nausea, physical weakness, and lack of coordination.

Description

Alcohol consumption varies with the individual, from occasional social drinking to the complex disorder of alcoholism, the chronic, excess ingestion of and dependence upon alcohol to the point that it disrupts normal functioning.

Western Treatment

Black coffee and taking cold showers are well known home remedies for inebriation and for hangover symptoms. Western doctors advise alcoholics to seek professional help as soon as possible. The most successful kind of help involves working toward recovery or abstinence through group therapy (such as in Alcoholics Anonymous) or individual counseling. As for the more specific issue of hangovers, the best general advice is to rest, drink plenty of fluids, and take aspirin or some other painkiller to alleviate headache symptoms.

Western physicians sometimes prescribe medications to treat the physical complications of alcoholism, such as ulcers. Hospitalization may be necessary in some cases of severe physical damage or withdrawal symptoms such as delirium tremens. Following the patient's withdrawal from alcohol, Western doctors sometimes prescribe the drug Antabuse to render the person more sensitive to alcohol and thus more likely to experience a very unpleasant, off-putting reaction to drinking it.

144

Chinese Treatment

Like their Western counterparts, Chinese doctors advise alcoholics to get professional help as soon as possible, preferably in the form of group or individual counseling. Many substance abuse programs successfully treat alcoholism and other dependencies with ear acupuncture, which is difficult to do at home.

For treating a hangover, I recommend the following steps:
- Pinch hard on LR 1 and N 1.
- Massage GB 8 to alleviate headache and vomiting caused by excessive alcohol.
- Massage LI 4, DU 22, LR 2, and LR 8.
- Massage micromeridian N: palm side of fifth finger, the channel next to the fourth finger, from the tip to the palm.
- Between drinking sessions, tonify body systems and reduce the craving for alcohol by means of these actions:
  - Massage LR 3 and micromeridian N (see above) to tonify the Liver.
  - Massage HT 7 to decrease the craving.
  - Avoid sour foods.

Anorexia (Anorexia Nervosa)
(also see *Bulimia*)

Symptoms

The clearest behaviors associated with anorexia are a severe restriction of food intake and an overall preoccupation with food and meals. Sometimes periods of sparse eating alternate with periods of bingeing on food, followed by self-induced vomiting or, with the help of laxatives, quick defecation to avoid weight gain (see *Bulimia* in this guide). Often anorexics exercise a lot to burn off even more body weight.

The results of anorexia include rapid weight loss and thinness, possibly accompanied by menstrual irregularities or lack of menstruation in women; insomnia; dental problems; cold intolerance (occasionally with blueness and numbness of the hands and feet); and/or skin changes, such as peeling.

Description

Many factors can lead a person to engage in behaviors that cause anorexia nervosa, which, like bulimia, is a widespread eating disorder. One of the strongest is the cultural pressure to be physically slim and, therefore, sexually attractive. This pressure is imposed more heavily upon women than men, which accounts for why anorexia is more common among women.

Teenage girls are especially inclined toward anorexic behavior. Physiologically, they are already undergoing major changes in body appearance due to hormonal shifts. Given this fact and the cultural emphasis on slimness, they can become so insecure about how they are physically evolving that they can't judge the matter rationally; they continue to see themselves as fat—even in a mirror—regardless of how thin they become.

Psychologically, teenage girls are just beginning to cope not only with their rapidly maturing bodies but also with the escalating challenges of adulthood, including dating and making more serious academic, work, and lifestyle choices. Under the emotional strain of all this coping, they may resort to anorexic behavior as at least one means of having firm control over their lives.

According to Western medicine, other major or contributing causes of anorexia may be a family history of depression or alcoholism (another form of food-related addiction) and hormonal or neuroendocrine disturbances (possibly related to the hypothalamus, which regulates many physiological functions such as appetite, sleep, and sexual behavior).

Chinese medicine also regards anorexia as a complex illness involving both physical and emotional systems. In addition, it maintains the following facts:

- The depression leading to and/or fueling anorexia may be caused by a Lung Qi or a Liver Qi disharmony.

146

- The underlying fear among anorexics of not being attractive or acceptable may be associated with an imbalance of Kidney Qi.
- An anorexic's craving for attractiveness or acceptance may be linked to a disturbance of Heart Qi. Whatever the case, Heart Qi is going to be adversely affected by any emotional turmoil, including the kind associated with anorexia.
- Spleen Qi, which facilitates digestion, is disturbed by the dietary extremes that an anorexic practices.

Western Treatment

If you suspect anorexia, it is important to consult a physician as soon as possible. The best treatment plan consists of a team approach: at least one family member or friend to offer emotional support and to help guarantee healthy dietary and lifestyle practices at home; a physician; a psychotherapist; a nutritionist; and possibly a dentist. In some cases, antidepressant medication may be helpful. For more information, contact:

The American Anorexia/Bulimia Association
133 Cedar Lane
Teaneck, NJ 07666
(201) 836-1800

National Association of Anorexia Nervosa
    and Associated Disorders
Box 271
Hyde Park, IL 60035
(312) 831-3438

Chinese Treatment

In addition to pursuing the Western treatment, do the following to help balance all aspects of energetic disturbance:
- Consult *Emotional Problems* in this guide, determine which energy channel is most out of balance, and treat it accordingly.

- Massage CV 12 and SP 9 to improve Digestive Qi.
- Massage SP 15: good for any depression associated with an eating disorder.
- For fear associated with anorexia, massage the following points:

  BL 23 and BL 52; or, alternatively, massage the lower back in a large, circular, clockwise manner to include the outer BL points.

  KI 1, KI 4, and KI 6.
- For vomiting associated with anorexia, massage P 6 immediately after eating and CV 9 anytime after eating.
- To calm the Heart, massage HT 5, HT 7, and P 6.
- To restore harmony to the hypothalamus gland, massage GB 8.

Appetite, Poor

Symptoms

Lack of interest in eating, possibly accompanied by any of the following symptoms: perceived loss of taste; distended, gaseous abdomen; fatigue; loose stool after eating; dry mouth; constipation; vomiting after forcing self to eat.

Description

Western medicine explains appetite as a perception of being hungry or full that's controlled by the brain's hypothalamus gland, usually in accordance with a person's physical need for nourishment. Appetite also can be psychologically driven, when the emotional need to eat—or not eat, as with eating disorders— overrides the physical one. Infections, chronic illnesses, and drug use, especially amphetamines, also can lead to loss of appetite.

In Chinese medicine, a lack of appetite is due to some disturbance in the Digestive Qi channels—that is, the SP and Stomach channels. Aside from a general treatment to stimulate these channels, more specific treatments can more directly address specific symptoms (see the Chinese treatment below).

Western Treatment

Prescription medications can stimulate appetite. At home, treatments include more definite mealtimes (no snacks), more attention to preparing well-balanced meals that the person likes, and making sure that the dining experience is restful and aesthetically pleasing.

Chinese Treatment

As a general treatment in all cases, massage the following:
* SP 6
* F micromeridian on hand, from tip to palm
* the midback, in clockwise fashion

For more specific treatment, choose the description that best fits the particular situation and add the designated massage points or areas:
* If food has no taste, or if there's a refusal to eat, no interest in food, or a distended, gaseous abdomen: add LI 4 and ST 44.
* If there's vomiting after forcing oneself to eat, some abdominal distension: add LI 11 and ST 36.
* If there's no desire for eating, loose stool after eating, or fatigue: add massaging the lower abdomen and the lower back in a clockwise direction.
* If there's dry mouth, drinking but no eating, or constipation: add KI 3, ST 36, and ST 44.

Asthma

Symptoms

Wheezing, shortness of breath, rapid breathing, prolonged expiration, bluish lips (or "cyanosis," due to lack of oxygen).

Description

Western medicine still does not completely understand how asthma develops. It is characterized by a constriction (narrowing) of the airways that's apparently brought on by allergens in the environment, infectious agents, and/or a strong emotional reaction. The constriction is partly due to greater mucus secretion, which results in blocked airways and breathing difficulty. As air squeezes through smaller airways, it makes a wheezing sound. The narrower the airways become, the louder the wheeze and the harder the breathing. When the airway is completely blocked, no air goes through, and breathing is very labored with no wheezing.

Consult a physician at the first sign of possible asthma. Usually it can be diagnosed with a physical examination alone, but a chest X ray, blood test, blood gas level check, and/or allergy testing also may be necessary.

Chinese medicine defines asthma as a disturbance in the flow of Lung Qi. It is important to understand the role of Lung Qi to appreciate how Chinese medicine accounts for and treats the development of asthma.

The Lung itself is closely connected to the skin through the spreading of Qi. Lung Qi is involved in the formation of Qi from the air and in the movement of Qi throughout the body. The Qi layer formed in the skin and the superficial parts of the body under the skin fends off invasion by external pathogens. In this way it acts like a protective shield over the body and is partially analogous to what Western medicine perceives as the immune system. A weakness in Defensive Qi—which, among other things, might lead to asthma—can be caused by a number of factors, including heredity, prenatal injury, drug or alcohol use, smoking, physical illness, improper diet, and/or emotional stress.

Whatever the cause, the weakened Defensive Qi system becomes vulnerable to Wind—a Chinese concept that includes not only the natural wind but also everything that is carried by it, such as dust, pollen, dander, other allergens, virus, and bacteria. This Defensive Qi vulnerability, combined with a Kidney Qi weakness and a negative Wind impact, results in asthma: spasm in the airways and a reversal of Lung Qi that causes coughing and wheezing.

Western Treatment

There are two basic forms of treatment: maintaining one's health between attacks, and dealing with an acute attack. Each form is described separately below.

For health maintenance between attacks, take prescribed medication or medications to prevent or at least delay the next attack. Possible prescribed medications include bronchodilators (sometimes supplemented by steroids) to open airways for freer breathing, antibiotics to fight infectious agents, and/or allergy shots to boost immunity to specific allergens. Instead of, or in addition to, taking allergy shots, it may be advisable to avoid certain known or potential sources of allergens.

For an acute attack, take the prescribed medication or medications and increase intake of fluids to loosen phlegm and mucus. If breathing is severely difficult, visit a hospital emergency room for intravenous therapy.

Chinese Treatment

There are two basic forms of treatment. The first is maintaining a state of good health between attacks: Chinese physicians believe in the ancient saying "Winter disease, Summer cure," which means that giving treatment when there are no symptoms (Summer) helps prevent illness later (Winter). The second form of treatment is dealing with an acute attack.

For health maintenance between attacks, strengthen the Lung and Kidney systems by massaging the following areas (can be used along with taking prescribed medications):
  * upper back in a circular, clockwise motion, to tonify the Lungs and calm the mind

151

- lower back in a circular, clockwise motion, to tonify the Kidneys
- midback in a circular, clockwise motion, to strengthen the digestive systems and decrease the formation of phlegm
- the BL lines from the shoulder down to the hip
- BL 13
- LU 9, the source point on the Lung channel, which is located at a dent or hole that can be felt below the thumb at the wrist crease
- the "chest area" on each hand: on the middle finger—the section closest to the palm
- the micromeridian C, which corresponds to the Lung channel, massage both hands: always starting at the base of the fourth finger (palm side) and going toward the tip, without going backward (which would be *against* the normal flow of Qi)

These activities help to open blocked channels and restore the healthy flow of Qi and air. They also assist fluid movement, so that the excess mucus blocking the airways becomes thinner. Massage on a daily basis to lengthen the period between attacks.

Also, avoid foods that generate phlegm: dairy products, sugar, honey, peanuts, almonds, or pork. Choose foods that tend to thin phlegm: mushrooms, papaya, potatoes, pumpkin, radishes, strawberries, or string beans. If the phlegm is thick and yellow (known as "hot" phlegm), white fungus is the most healing food. If it's not available, choose asparagus, apples, carrots, celery, pears, or mangoes, and avoid hot foods such as garlic and ginger.

Finally, refrain from excess physical or mental activity—whether it's work or recreation. Also remember that maintaining your emotional equilibrium is very important to your health in general and to managing asthma in particular. Avoid stressful situations and emotional outbursts such as overt displays of anger or frustration. Some form of meditation or therapy may help in this endeavor. Massaging the following points also can be calming: HT 7 and CV 15.

Under the supervision of a Western and a Chinese physician,

you may be able to decrease the dosage of medication gradually over time as you continue to administer acupressure and eat the proper foods.

For an acute attack, immediately and vigorously stimulate the following:

- Ding Chuan, an "extra point" for asthma. The phrase means "stop wheeze." It actually consists of two points, located on the back of the neck directly below and to the sides of the biggest bump on the spine.
- GB 20, the Wind Gate at the back of the neck: the bump halfway between the ear and the middle of the neck
- GB 21
- LU 9
- CV 17
- the upper back, in a circular, clockwise motion
- BL13

Also, for a calming effect, massage HT 7 and CV 15.

Note: At least at first, be sure to perform acupressure in conjunction with prescribed medications. The quality of a person's response to acupressure during an acute attack depends on the severity of the asthma, the length of the illness, age, and general state of health. Younger and healthier people tend to have better responses.

If you find over time that the response to acupressure and proper diet is good (as evidenced by a diminished need for use of inhalers), you can then try acupressure without medication for the next *mild* attack.

It is important to remember that medication often works faster in an acute situation, while acupressure does more over time to tonify the body and help prevent further attacks.

Consult a physician to get a proper diagnosis when you first suspect asthma. Consult a physician immediately when a severe attack occurs. If a physician is not available at that time, go to a hospital emergency room.

Attention Deficit Disorder
(ADHD, ADD)

Symptoms

ADHD is the more recent term for the well-known condition called ADD, which has numerous symptoms grouped by Western medicine into three main categories below. Any single case of ADD involves multiple symptoms from these categories:

1. *inattentiveness:* includes (among other symptoms) failing to pay close attention to details and making careless mistakes; difficulty sustaining attention in tasks or activities; appearance of not listening when spoken to directly
2. *hyperactivity:* includes (among other symptoms) fidgeting with hands or feet or squirming in seat; difficulty engaging in leisure activities quietly; excessive talking
3. *impulsiveness:* includes (among other symptoms) often interrupting others and difficulty taking turns

In addition, numerous associated impairments may be present in the person's day-to-day functioning, such as:

* poor overall academic performance at school (7 to 15 points below on standardized tests)
* learning disabilities affecting reading and math
* memory problems
* speech and language difficulties
* trouble following rules or directions
* difficulty making plans or learning from experience
* impaired awareness of time
* low level of creativity or self-motivation
* sensory problems, especially relating to hearing
* problems in physical coordination and movement
* sleep-related problems

There also may be emotional problems, such as depression, anxiety, or other psychiatric or mood disorders.

Description

In Western terms, ADD is a very complex condition that affects every aspect of the person's life: physical, emotional, mental, and social. The precise cause is still undetermined, but most Western experts believe it is caused by defects in the neurological structure or pathways of the brain, or by a disorder in the brain chemicals called neurotransmitters. Recently two genes have been identified that may be connected to ADD.

ADD is currently the most common neurodevelopmental disorder of childhood. Recently the diagnosis has been extended to include children as young as age three. Approximately 5 to 10 percent of school-age children carry the diagnosis. It often continues into adulthood.

In Chinese terms, ADD is the result of disharmony in many energetic channels, the two most frequently affected being the Liver and Heart channels. It also can be attributed to an inherited tendency (which corresponds to the Western notion of a genetic link). The basis of this disharmony may involve Kidney Qi, because Kidney Yin is the foundation for all Yin (essence, fluid, blood) in the body, and Kidney Yang is the foundation for all Yang (fire).

The Kidney in Chinese medicine is the organ associated with ancestral inheritance, which means that ADD may be caused at least in part by a Kidney weakness passed down through the generations. This corresponds to the Western discovery of a possible genetic link.

Liver Yin is the home of an individual's Ethereal Soul, which is closely connected to his or her Mind (see the entry *Emotional Problems*). Therefore, when Liver Yin is disturbed, the Mind doesn't function well, which accounts for the symptoms of impulsivity, inattentiveness, and difficulty learning. The Mind also is closely connected with the Heart and, as a result, vulnerable to both physical and emotional manifestations of Heart disharmonies. In addition, the emotion of anger is associated with Liver and Heart imbalances, which would explain the symptoms of irritability, frustration, and even rage that are common among ADD sufferers.

Another factor in the development of ADD can be gastrointestinal or dietary influences. An accumulation of phlegm when Spleen energy is weak may result in a "misting" of the Mind, which then doesn't function well.

Western Treatment

It is advisable to consult a medical doctor as soon as ADD or ADHD is suspected. Treatment generally involves medication: stimulants (such as Ritalin or Dexedrine) or antidepressants (such as Imipramine, Norpramaine, or Prozac). It is important to know that such medications can have significant side effects; discuss this matter with the doctor. Treatment also can include psychotherapy or some form of behavioral or cognitive therapy.

Chinese Treatment

Currently there is no widely used Chinese medical treatment program for ADD, a disorder that is relatively recent even for Western medicine. The specific guidelines here are based on my own extensive research into ADD and my years of experience in working with ADD-affected individuals.

Like Western treatment, Chinese treatment needs to be multifaceted, as the guidelines below indicate. Also like Western treatment, it may take some time before you see any results. In my experience, the younger the person is, the better the response to treatment. Children under age seven usually respond the best.

I've found that using Chinese acupuncture, dietary and herbal regimens, combined with a home treatment program complement medication-based Western treatment and often work to decrease the amount of medication a person needs, which reduces the risk or intensity of unwanted side effects. For this reason and others, Chinese treatment is most effective when it's supervised by a medical doctor who is also an acupuncturist or by a medical doctor and an acupuncturist working together. Under these circumstances, the tapering of medication can be managed in close, timely coordination with acupuncture treatment and the type of home therapy outlined below.

To help alleviate any case of ADD or ADHD, do the following at home:

- Massage HT 7 to calm the Heart.
- Massage LR 3 and KI 6 *together* (at the same time or in alternating sequence).
- Massage the back Shu points—on both sides of the spine, from the shoulder down to the hips, to harmonize the Qi flow to all organs.
- Massage DU 20 and A 33 to assist mental concentration: for a child, just before homework; for an adult, just before a particularly demanding task or meeting.
- Massage the upper back in a clockwise direction to alleviate explosive anger or lack of focus and concentration.
- Massage the middle back in a clockwise direction to help prevent forgetfulness.
- Massage the lower back (Kidney area) in a clockwise direction if there's a history of ADD in the family, especially involving immediate family members.
- Eliminate phlegm-producing and hot foods from the diet. Also avoid excessive intake of cold foods, sour foods (such as pickles), and bitter foods (such as bitter chocolate).
- Incorporate meditation or some other form of gentle relaxation into the person's daily lifestyle.

Baldness (or Hair Loss)

Symptoms

Loss of head hair in patches or across the entire scalp; may be gradual or rapid, depending on the cause.

Description

The most common cause of baldness among men and women is aging. For men, a hereditary predisposition toward baldness is often a factor. It commonly begins during a man's thirties and gradually increases as he ages. In some cases this type of baldness begins even earlier. Usually it progresses in a pattern, with partial hair loss in specific areas, such as the crown of the head and/or the temples (a phenomenon known as "male pattern baldness"). For women, baldness due to aging tends to begin around menopause, with gradual thinning of the hair across the scalp.

Other causes of baldness, especially rapidly progressing baldness at any age, are scalp infections (most often fungal, but sometimes bacterial); chronic, debilitating diseases; chemotherapy; and radiation therapy.

Chinese medicine relates baldness to a decline or depletion of Kidney Essense, which nourishes the hair and gives it health, good color, and thickness. Kidney Essence is influenced by heredity, youth, lifestyle, diet, and general health.

Treatment of baldness aims at preventing the loss of inherited Kidney Essence and increasing the supply of postnatal (noninherited) Kidney Essence, mainly through Essence-containing food. Among the lifestyle factors that contribute to a premature loss of Kidney Essence in men is excessive sexual activity, because the Essence is lost through ejaculation. Chinese and Western medicine agree that once baldness has occurred in a given area, it is difficult if not impossible to trigger new hair growth there.

Western Treatment

To stimulate hair follicles and, therefore, help retard or minimize baldness due to aging, regular shampooing and scalp massage are recommended. It's also advisable to avoid using chemical preparations on the hair and to minimize wearing tight hats.

To counteract baldness-producing infections, various anti-fungal or antibiotic medications can be prescribed. To treat baldness for cosmetic purposes, hair transplants or certain drugs (e.g., Minoxidil) can be used, but the results are often unsatisfactory.

Chinese Treatment

To help prevent or retard the progression of baldness due to aging or other causes, do the following:

- Massage KI 3, KI 7, and the lower back (in a clockwise direction).
- Decrease stress and (for men) sexual activity.
- Increase consumption of Essence-containing foods (see food list).
- Do Qigong or Tai Chi exercises, which can help tonify the Kidneys.

Bedwetting (Enuresis)

Symptoms

Light or heavy involuntary urination while sleeping, possibly accompanied by any of the following symptoms: pale complexion, red cheeks, increased frequency or amount of urination during the day, poor appetite, weak limbs, emotional difficulties, yellowish discharge from the urethra or vagina.

Description

Bedwetting is common among young children and generally is not diagnosed as an illness (enuresis) unless it occurs after age eight. It chronically or periodically effects 15 to 30 percent of school-age children and in some cases persists into adulthood. There are two major types of enuresis: primary nocturnal enuresis (PNE), when the person has never been dry at night or has never been been dry for more than one year; and secondary nocturnal enuresis (SNE), when the person has had a history of being dry at night for at least one year.

Western science does not yet fully understand why or how enuresis develops. Multiple factors may interplay, including genetic makeup, psychological predispositions, sleeping disorders, and abnormalities in the urinary reservoir or in urinary production. Although enuresis itself doesn't cause physical harm, treatment is advisable because of the inconvenience associated with it and the adverse social and psychological effects it can have on the person and his or her family members.

In Chinese terms, all bedwetting is due to a Qi deficiency. What is called PNE in Western terms is a Kidney Qi deficiency associated with coldness. The person is unable to control urine flow, and bedwetting is usually marked by a large volume of urine, so that the sheets and body are soaked in the morning. The person's complexion is often pale. During the daytime there may be a lot of urine, usually clear. Emotionally the person may be insecure and fearful. The voice may be low-pitched, and the hands and feet may feel cold all the time.

In Chinese medicine, the disorder called SNE in Western terms indicates that the body is recuperating poorly or incompletely after one or more illnesses, or that other health problems are causing weakness in the digestive system, Kidneys, and Bladder. The Digestive Qi is low, and fluid accumulates. The urine discharged at night is usually small in volume, while during the day there may be an increased frequency of urination with a small amount each time. Other symptoms include pale face, weak spirit, weak limbs, poor appetite, and little thirst. There may even be coughing or other respiratory problems.

In addition to PNE and SNE, Chinese medicine recognizes a third kind of enuresis associated with emotional difficulties and infections of the urethra/bladder or vagina. The possible symptoms include red cheeks, yellowish discharge from the urethra or vagina, emotional irritability or agitation (which may result in bedwetting to get attention), and sleeptalking.

Western Treatment

The first-choice treatment is usually some kind of prescribed alarm that wakes the person just before, or at the onset of, nocturnal urination. A second-choice treatment is prescribed medication. A disadvantage of the latter treatment is a high regression rate and the possibility of negative side effects.

Chinese Treatment

To provide general restoration of Qi energy and, as a result, lessen the chance of bedwetting, massage CV 3 and SP 6.

To alleviate PNE, massage the following:
* KI 3 and KI 7
* the lower back, in a clockwise direction
* the J micromeridian on the hand that corresponds to the Kidney channel and is located on the back and side of the fifth finger; massage from the tip toward the palm

Also, keep the abdomen warm, avoid excessive intake of salty foods, and avoid being chilled in general—for example, dress warmly during cold weather.

To alleviate SNE, massage the following:
* SP 6 and LU 7
* the upper and middle back, in a clockwise direction
* the F micromeridian on the middle of the fifth finger, palm side, from the tip toward the palm
* the C micromeridian that corresponds to the Lung channel and is located on the palm side of the fourth finger next to the third finger; massage from the palm to the tip

Also, avoid excess intake of sweet foods, which can weaken the digestive system.

To alleviate the third type of enuresis associated with emotional upset, do the following:
* Massage LR 3, LR 8, and HT 7.

- Avoid excessive intake of sour or bitter foods (such as pickles or bitter chocolate).
- Teach the person breathing exercises and other means of self-calming.

Belching (Excessive)

Symptoms

Sharp, noisy release of air from the stomach through the mouth, often accompanied by distention of the stomach.

Description

Belching is usually the result of swallowing excessive air, which then seeks a quick release. Often this swallowing occurs while eating. Other causes include gum-chewing, excessive intake of carbonated beverages, smoking, or anxiety. Most cases of chronic belching can be attributed to emotional problems that lead to an increase in air-swallowing.

In terms of Chinese medicine, the Stomach is responsible for moving food and other stomach contents—including air—downward. When excess air is swallowed, the Stomach swells, there is an uncomfortable feeling of fullness, and Stomach Qi "rebels." This results in belching: air movement in the opposite direction. Chinese medicine also maintains that emotions can play a substantial role in chronic belching.

Western Treatment

No treatment exists for isolated episodes of belching after meals. For chronic belching, it's advisable to reduce air swallowing by chewing food instead of gulping it, eating and drinking slowly, avoiding chewing gum, and clenching a pencil between the teeth. It may also be wise to seek counseling for possible emotional problems.

Chinese Treatment

To regulate Lung Qi and Stomach Qi and calm the emotions, massage LU 9, ST 36, ST 43, and LR 5. To alleviate stomach distention and an uncomfortable feeling of fullness, also massage ST 41.

Bladder Infection (Urinary Cystitis)

Symptoms

Burning sensation or pain with urination; increased frequency of urination; increased pressure to urinate; cloudy or bloody urine.

Description

Western medicine attributes most cases of bladder infection to bacteria coming up from the urethra. Aside from inflaming the bladder, the infectious bacteria may reach upward toward the kidney. Anatomical abnormalities along this route can contribute to the risk or extent of infection, as can holding back urine for an excessive period of time (e.g., children delaying urination while playing, or adults while working).

Chinese medicine diagnoses bladder infection in a similar way, but the terminology differs. According to the Chinese system, the cause is excessive damp heat in the bladder, which relates to the Western concept of a bacterial infection causing systemic "heat" (fever) or localized "heat" in that region of the body. The dampness translates into thickened urine (in Western terms, infected urine "thickened" with many white cells).

Western Treatment

Increase fluid intake, and avoid holding back urine. Also keep the genital area clean. An acute episode of bladder infection may be treated with a short course of antibiotics. A chronic condition is often treated with maintenance antibiotics between active infections to prevent or postpone recurrence. Kidney infections are much more serious than bladder infections and sometimes require hospitalization for intravenous (IV) therapy.

Chinese Treatment

To resolve the dampness, clear the heat, and stimulate urination, do the following:

- Increase fluid intake, and empty the bladder whenever it feels full.
- Massage SP 9, SP 6, ST 40, BL 20, BL 22, BL 28, CV 3, and BL 63.
- Massage the lower back, including the outer BL line, in a clockwise fashion.
- Massage the I micromerdian middle of the fifth finger, backhand side, from the hand toward the tip.
- Avoid coldness to the lower back and the lower abdomen.
- Avoid excess intake of cold and hot foods.

Bleeding, External

(see *Bleeding, Internal* for bleeding related to ulcers
or internal hemorrhages, coughing up or vomiting blood,
or blood in the urine or stool)

Symptoms

Blood flowing, oozing, or, if an artery is involved, spurting from a cut, break, or scrape in the skin

Description

The most common cause of a cut, break, or scrape in the skin that results in external bleeding is trauma—in other words, a sudden blow, fall, or abrasion that damages the skin and possibly internal structures. Normally the blood soon clots and the bleeding stops. Bleeding continues if clotting doesn't occur, which may be due to hemorrhaging (large amounts of blood seeping through the blood vessel walls); a blood condition such as hemophilia; or another cause of bleeding that is not being treated, such as a deeper wound. Severe bleeding—loss of more than a quart—can lead to shock or even death. Mild, chronic bleeding can result in anemia.

Other causes of external bleeding are menstruation (see *Menstrual Problems* in this guide), which occurs normally in non-menopausal women once a month, or a skin condition that produces open or easily punctured sores. For coping with bleeding from a skin condition, first establish what the condition is, then follow the appropriate treatment guidelines.

Chinese medicine acknowledges these causes, but also considers the Spleen to be responsible for "holding" blood within the blood vessels and, in general, keeping blood in its place.

Western Treatment

Apply pressure directly to the area of bleeding, and elevate the bleeding part of the body (e.g., the leg if the bleeding wound is on the leg). If possible, apply ice to the area of bleeding; the cold will cause constriction of the blood vessels, which will help reduce the volume of blood.

It is best *not* to apply a tourniquet above the bleeding area because the pressure will cut off the blood supply to the entire area below. This could result in a need to amputate all or part of that area. If the caregiver is knowledgeable about first aid and if the bleeding comes from an artery, he or she may be able to apply pressure just to the artery itself, which is the most effective treatment (e.g., pressing on the brachial artery on the inside of the arm to stop bleeding from that area).

Chinese Treatment

In addition to the Western treatment guidelines above, do the following:

- Pinch SP 1 very hard to give it strong stimulation. In cases of minor bleeding, this can help stop the flow. In cases of major hemorrhaging, it may help decrease the flow.

165

- Pinch F 1 (the point on the hand that corresponds to SP 1), located at the middle of the tip of the little finger.

Bleeding, Internal

Symptoms

Depending on the situation, any of the following: coughing or vomiting blood; blood in the urine or stool; bleeding from the rectum or any other body orifice.

Description

Internal bleeding most often results from a damaged or diseased organ or area of tissue within the body (e.g., an ulcer in the stomach or a tumor in the colon).

Chinese medicine agrees with this description, but also maintains that the Spleen is responsible for "holding" blood within the blood vessels and, in general, keeping blood in its place.

Western Treatment

Seek professional guidance, as appropriate. A small amount of internal bleeding usually represents a nonemergency situation but warrants medical testing to determine the cause. A large amount, indicating a hemorrhage, represents an emergency situation that may require transfusion and/or surgery.

Chinese Treatment

Follow the guidelines above (see "Western treatment"), and also do the following:
- Pinch SP 1 very hard to give it strong stimulation. In cases of minor bleeding, this can help stop the flow. In cases of major hemorrhaging, it may help decrease the flow.
- Pinch F 1 (the point on the hand that corresponds to SP 1), located at the middle of the tip of the little finger.

Bruises

Symptoms

Suddenly appearing colored spots on the skin that may or may not be painful to the touch and that change color over time.

Description

Bruises occur when small blood vessels (capillaries) are injured and rupture. Blood leaks out of the vessels into the surrounding tissue, causing pain, swelling, and a bluish-purplish discoloration of the skin. Bruises heal gradually as the blood leaked into the tissue is broken down and reabsorbed into the nearby blood and lymphatic vessels.

Chinese medicine offers a similar description of bruises, identifying them as external manifestations of "blood stasis," which includes internal clotting.

Western Treatment

Apply ice or some other cold object to the injured area immediately following trauma. This action constricts the blood vessels and decreases the oozing of blood into the surrounding tissue. Small bruises, especially those that occur on the arms or legs, generally heal on their own without needing medical attention.

Under the following circumstances it is important to seek professional evaluation:
- when the injury is severe and the resulting bruise is large and very painful
- when there is significant trauma to the chest or abdomen
- when the bruise is causing swelling of the eyes
- when the bruise is very large on the face or forehead
- when the bruise occurs spontaneously, without any related injury
- when the bruise does not heal after two weeks

Chinese Treatment

Consult a professional under the more serious circumstances listed above (see "Western Treatment"). To assist in healing smaller bruises, do the following, as appropriate:

- For all bruises: massage SP 10 and BL 17, and massage around the bruise itself in a circular, clockwise fashion (the "turtle" technique).
- For a shoulder-area bruise: massage LI 16.

Bulimia
(also see *Anorexia*)

Symptoms

Binge eating, usually of high-calorie foods, that is often done quickly and secretly, followed by self-induced vomiting or quick, laxative-driven defecation to avoid weight gain; may be accompanied by depression.

Description

Bulimia, along with anorexia, is a widespread eating disorder that can have multiple physical and emotional causes. It is often associated with a culturally induced desire to be thin and, therefore, sexually attractive. Other causes include a family history of depression or alcoholism (a similar form of self-destructive behavior) and, possibly, hormonal and neuroendocrine disturbances due to poor functioning of the hypothalamus gland, which regulates hunger, appetite, sleep, and sexual behavior.

Unlike anorexia, which is more typical of teenagers and results in their starving themselves to the point of extreme thinness, bulimia tends to affect women in their early twenties and produce more moderate results. In many cases the body continues to appear normal in weight, and professional help isn't sought until the bulimic is in her thirties. Many bulimics also engage in other impulsive, self-destructive behaviors, such as alcoholism or drug abuse. Among the possible medical consequences of bulimia are potassium depletion and dental problems caused by stomach acid.

Western Treatment

If you suspect bulimia, consult a medical doctor immediately. The most effective treatment strategy is a team approach: at least one family member or friend to offer emotional support and to help guarantee healthy dietary and lifestyle practices at home; a physician; a psychotherapist; a nutritionist; and possibly a dentist. In some situations antidepressant medication may be advised. For more information, contact:

The American Anorexia/Bulimia Association
133 Cedar Lane
Teaneck, NJ 07666
(201) 836-1800

National Association of Anorexia Nervosa
  and Associated Disorders
Box 271
Hyde Park, IL 60035
(312) 831-3438

Chinese Treatment

Besides the above measures (see "Western Treatment"), do the following things to help balance all aspects of energetic disturbance:

- Massage ST 36, SP 6, and LI 11 regularly.
- Tonify the F micromeridan on the hand: massage the middle of the little finger, from the tip toward the palm.
- For vomiting associated with bulimia, massage CV 9 and CV 16 anytime after eating.
- To calm the Heart, massage HT 5, HT 7, and P 6.

- To restore harmony to the hypothalamus gland, massage GB 8.
- To alleviate depression, massage SP 15.

Cold, Common

Symptoms

Combinations of the following: runny nose, sore throat, sneezing, stuffy nose, tightness in the chest, watery eyes, and sometimes fever or body aches.

Description

In Western terms the common cold is caused by a virus, usually an airborne one that's inhaled. In some cases a common cold may be part of an overall case of influenza ("the flu").

A common cold can be a serious disorder in infants and young children because of the immaturity of their immune systems. For example, a two-week-old baby with a cold may require hospitalization. In general, colds become less frequent and less serious as the individual matures. On average, preschoolers catch ten to twelve colds a year, with ear infection being the most frequent complication. School-age children typically miss school about five times a year due to colds, with one or two possible bouts in the summer.

Most colds last less than a week, but sometimes symptoms may linger for as long as two weeks, especially for adults. People who have chronic illnesses are more susceptible to colds as a result of their weakened immune systems.

Chinese medicine does not dispute the existence of cold viruses but believes that environmental influences, such as wet feet or overexposure to cold air, can contribute to the illness. The Chinese explanation relates well to the Western concept of catching a cold due to bad weather: the body uses up Defensive Qi (Wei Qi), which circulates close to the skin, to combat harmful, incoming Wind elements and, in so doing, renders itself more susceptible to invasion from what Westerners call viruses. In four-season climates, colds are more frequent during the winter and spring because temperatures change more radically at these times of year.

Perverse Wind elements can enter the body through the nose, mouth, or pores of the skin to disrupt the circulation of Defensive Qi. Because Chinese medicine posits that the skin is closely connected to the Lungs and the nasal passages, whatever enters the skin can lead directly to the respiratory system and result in a congested or runny nose, coughing, and possibly fever. Children are more vulnerable to colds because their skin is considered "tender," which means that the pores are widely open, Defensive Qi circulation is more compromised, and immunity against external pathogens is weaker.

The Chinese recognize two different types of cold-producing agents: Wind Cold and Wind Heat (which could correspond to what Westerners known as viral and bacterial infections, respectively). Here are the specific symptoms associated with each kind:

- *Wind Cold:* strong dislike of cold, sneezing, clear nasal discharge or thin phlegm, mild sore throat, cough
- *Wind Heat:* mild dislike of cold, high fever, sweating, thick nasal discharge or cough with thick phlegm, painful sore throat, dry mouth, red face, body aches

A Wind Cold illness is generally milder than a Wind Heat one, which is analogous to a viral infection usually being less troublesome than a bacterial one. A Wind Cold attack can, however, weaken the body so that a more serious Wind Heat invasion takes place. A single, prolonged case of Wind Cold or repeated cases over a short time period can depress Lung Qi, resulting in more phlegm formation and possibly the complications known in Western medicine as bronchitis or pneumonia, which are often characterized by a very phlegm-producing cough.

Western Treatment

Decrease physical activity and increase bed rest to avoid exhaustion and body strain. Also, drink plenty of liquids and use a humidifier to loosen mucus and prevent dehydration. Commercial medications may be used as directed to treat symptoms: aspirin (or other pain relievers) to relieve achiness and bring down fever; antihistamines to reduce sneezing and watery eyes; decongestants to relieve stuffy nose and tightness in the chest; and various syrups and drops to alleviate throat soreness and moderate coughing. Some multi-ingredient cold products combine several of these medications.

Chinese Treatment

At the onset of the illness, use acupressure to strengthen key points where Wind enters the body (see below). This treatment can be especially beneficial if you suspect exposure to a cold before any symptoms have appeared—for example, if you notice your child's playmate has a cold, or if your coworker has a cold. Also at the onset, determine whether it's a Wind Cold or a Wind Heat type, according to the criteria listed above.

For colds in general—both Wind Cold and Wind Heat types—the treatment consists of "clearing the Wind" and then relieving the symptoms. For either type, massage the following points and body areas:

- LI 4, the "head point," found in the web between the thumb and the index finger, to treat/prevent headaches, nasal congestion, and sore throat
- GB 20, the main "Wind Gate" at the back of the neck—the bump halfway between the ear and the middle of the neck; to clear harmful wind from the body
- ST 36, the "master immunity point" below the kneecap, on the outside face of the biggest bone, to strengthen Qi
- LU 7, and TB 5 to promote an even flow of interior heat
- DU 20 for generalized headache relief

- the upper back in a clockwise direction
- LI 20 to clear the nasal passages

For Wind Cold, do the following additional treatments:
- Cause sweating by taking a hot bath or hot shower, or by leaning the towel-draped head over a sink or a basin of hot water. Also place a humidifier by the bed so the steam comes toward it, and keep the body warm. Sweating opens the pores, drives out pathogens, and increases Defensive Qi circulation.

  Both Western medicine and Chinese medicine advise using a humidifier to treat the common cold. Both have found it to be effective in relieving symptoms, although for different reasons. Western medicine recommends it for providing extra moisture, through inhalation, to the lungs, thereby loosening thick mucus in the nose and chest. Chinese medicine recommends it for opening pores, which stimulates circulation of Defensive Qi.
- Also to cause sweating, massage LI 4 in a clockwise direction.
- Avoid cool or cold foods and foods that are iced or frozen.
- Increase intake of foods that are warm or hot to warm the body's interior and cause further sweating. For example, chicken soup cooked on low heat for a long time would be excellent.

For Wind Heat, do the following additional treatments:
- Cause a gradual decrease in body temperature with a luke-warm bath for twenty to thirty minutes. It should not be a cold bath, or it may cause shivering, which can adversely increase body temperature. Also, place a cool-air vaporizer by the bed so the vapor comes toward it. Western medicine also recommends using vaporizers to provide extra moisture.
- Increase intake of cool foods and liquids to cool down the body's interior. For example, chicken soup would not be appropriate, but apples and pears would. To decrease phlegm,

eat mushrooms, papaya, potatoes, pumpkin, radishes, straw-berries, and string beans.

- In addition to the general points mentioned above, also massage LI 11 to clear heat from the body, DU 14 to decrease fever, CV 17 to strengthen Qi flow to the chest, and LR 3 to alleviate body aches.
- Other points to massage, as appropriate, include HT 7 to calm the spirit (especially good for children who may become agitated by a high fever) and P 6 to overcome nausea and vomiting.

Consult a physician if symptoms last longer than a week without diminishing or if any of the following symptoms occur: persistent high fever, breathing trouble, earache, stiff neck, severely sore throat, or inability to drink liquids. If an antibiotic is prescribed, see appendix C for treating/avoiding side effects.

Cold Sores (or Mouth Ulcers)

Symptoms

Small, painful blisters (starting out as red pimples) on the lips and inside the mouth, usually occurring in clusters.

Description

In Western medicine, a cold sore is caused by a virus (herpes simplex type 1). It most commonly occurs in children from eight months to five years of age. Approximately 80 percent of adults have been infected with the herpes virus, and it can be found in the saliva of approximately 25 percent. Usually it spreads from person to person by direct contact and by sharing contaminated eating or drinking utensils.

The virus remains dormant in nerve cells and recurs with emotional or illness-related stress, such as a common cold. Most people notice a tingling sensation before cold sores break out at exactly the same place each time. The sores crust over within two to three days and go away in about ten to fourteen days.

In Chinese medicine, "cold" sores are actually considered "hot" Qi sores. They result from an accumulation of harmful heat, usually in the stomach or intestines due to overeating, especially foods that are greasy, fatty, fried, or hot and spicy. The heat flows upward to the mouth area and creates the sores. The same harmful heat also can be caused by toxins released from an infection.

There are two different types of cold sores, each with its own distinctive set of symptoms:

- *Excess type:* painful, shallow sores with bright red borders, possibly accompanied by a red tongue, red lips, fever, constipation, and/or thick urine
- *Deficiency type* (due to recurrent illnesses or stress causing fluid depletion and Qi deficiency in the Spleen and Kidney): chronic, deep sores that are dull red, possibly accompanied by red cheeks, restlessness, and/or thirst

Western Treatment

Often no treatment is given because cold sores go away by themselves in ten to fourteen days. For recurrent cold sores, a person can use over-the-counter lip balms or antiviral medications such as Acyclovir to relieve pain. The best approach to cold sores is prevention: avoid oral contact or the sharing of eating or drinking utensils with people who have cold sores. Also be aware of any possible emotional causes and do what you can to avoid triggering them. So far a vaccine is not available to keep a person from getting the virus.

Chinese Treatment

The same as in *Thrush* in this guide.

Colic

Symptoms

Colic usually occurs in infants three to four months of age. The baby cries suddenly and loudly, as if in pain. The abdomen becomes distended, the legs are often pulled up onto the abdomen, and the feet feel cold. The cry can last for minutes or even hours. Often the baby seems to feel better after passing gas or a stool.

Description

Colic remains a medical mystery. It affects an estimated 20 to 30 percent of infants under four months old and usually goes away on its own.

Western medicine offers many possible explanations for colic, all very general in kind, including developmental difficulties, unmet biological needs, stress from the parent-infant interaction, a built-in temperamental predisposition, or an overly agitated colon ("hypermotility" of the colon). Treatment is advisable not so much because of the condition itself but more because of the negative effect it can have on the parent-infant relationship.

In Chinese medicine, colic is due to indigestion resulting from a weakness in the Spleen or in Digestive Qi. The baby cannot digest milk or formula, so his or her Qi stagnates, and the abdomen accordingly becomes distended.

Western Treatment

Treatment is often directed at both the baby and the parents (especially the primary caregiver, if there is one, which usually is the mother). The parents need to develop coping or self-calming techniques to alleviate their own problems in tending an irritable, colicky baby. A change of formula or antispasmodic medications may be prescribed for the baby, but they are not always effective.

Chinese Treatment

Massage the following:

- the abdomen, clockwise in the direction of the large-intestine flow: up the right side (ascending colon), across the top (traverse colon), down the left side (descending colon), and back across the bottom to the right side again

- the F micromeridian on the middle of the fifth finger, palm side, from the tip to the palm
- when the baby appears frightened by colic, or is restless and cries a lot at night: the Yintang point between the eyebrows

Also, do the following:

- Do not overfeed the baby. When bottle-feeding, there may a tendency toward getting the baby to finish the bottle rather than letting the baby stop feeding on his or her own—the natural, self-limiting pattern associated with breast-feeding.
- Feed the baby on schedule rather than on demand. It will encourage a more regular duration of feeding and intake of food.
- If you're breast-feeding, avoid gas-producing and colic-aggravating foods, including beans, broccoli, brussels sprouts, cabbage, cauliflower, chocolate, citrus fruits, coffee, garlic, melons, onions, peaches, rhubarb, and tomatoes.
- Avoid cold foods.
- When the baby has a weak cry, cold hands and feet, and a pale face, a herbal remedy can help warm the intestines and works more effectively and naturally than antispasmodic medications: simply place a slice of ginger on the navel area. You can tape it down to keep it in place. Some authorities suggest preheating the ginger in a frying pan with some salt—just make sure it is not too hot when you apply it to the baby's skin. Leave it there for twenty minutes to an hour.

Conjunctivitis ("Pink Eye")

Symptoms

The whites of the eyes appear pink or even red; liquid discharge from the eyes; possibly swelling or itching of the eyes; runny nose.

Description

In Western terms, there are three common types of conjunctivitis, named according to their cause:

- *Allergic:* Usually the eyes are less red than they are with the other two types, although there may be added redness due to itchiness-related rubbing. The discharge is usually clear. There may be other allergic symptoms, such as a runny nose and skin rashes.
- *Viral:* The eyes are red and sometimes swollen, with clear or white discharge and, possibly, light sensitivity. This type may be a complication of a cold.
- *Bacterial:* This type is similar to the viral one, and also may be a complication of a cold, but the discharge from the eyes may be more yellow and puslike.

In Chinese terms, conjunctivitis is divided into two categories: acute (single-episode) and chronic (recurring episodes). An acute case is attributed to external pathogens or infectious agents. A chronic case may be the result of an internal Qi imbalance in the LR and GB meridians, both of which are connected to the eyes. This imbalance predisposes the eyes to become red and swollen.

Western Treatment

If you suspect conjunctivitis (any type), always consult a physician to make sure it's not something else, such as a foreign body in the eye, an abrasion from a contact lens, or a symptom of another, more serious condition such as acute glaucoma, herpes, or venereal disease. Newborn conjunctivitis (possibly due to gonorrhea or silver nitrate, which is routinely put in a newborn's eyes to prevent possible infection from the birth canal) should immediately be treated by a physician.

The most common treatments for conjunctivitis are as follows (according to type):

- *Allergic:* allergy eye drops, over-the-counter or prescription, and possibly an oral antihistamine; for severe cases, steroid drops. The duration of allergic conjunctivitis varies according to the duration of exposure. If you work outside and are allergic to pollen, you may need treatment during the entire blooming season. If you're allergic to a friend's cat, you may only need treatment while visiting that friend, or you may simply allow the conjunctivitis to resolve itself after you leave.
- *Bacterial* or *viral:* antibiotic eye drops or ointment; also, careful hand washing to prevent spreading the infection. Viral conjunctivitis usually is milder and goes away by itself after a few days. Bacterial conjunctivitis may be more severe. If left untreated, it can sometimes develop into a more serious eye infection.

Chinese Treatment

After consulting with a physician to rule out more serious causes of red eyes, do the following:

- For both acute and chronic: massage BL 1, GB 1, LI 4, and LI 11.
- For acute: add GB 20.
- For chronic: add LR 3.
- Physical considerations for chronic: to strengthen the LR and GB meridians, avoid excessive intake of sour and greasy foods and, specifically for the Liver's sake, avoid excess medication and alcohol.

Constipation

Symptoms

Infrequent defecation, often hard stools, sometimes accompanied by pain during defecation.

Description

In terms of Western medicine, constipation can be due to heredity, anatomical abnormalities, a low-fiber diet, or psychological predispositions (e.g., a tendency to become constipated when stressed). Normal frequency of defecation is considered to range from several times a day to once every few days, depending on the individual.

According to Chinese medicine, a healthy person should have a bowel movement every day. Several factors can interfere with this pattern to cause constipation:

- *Poor diet:* The major cause of constipation relates to improper food intake. An excess of cold foods contracts the intestines and slows down the normal movement of food through them. Alternatively, an excess of hot foods dries up the stools and makes them more difficult to excrete. As a result, they pile up in the large intestine.
- *Emotional stress:* The emotions of anger and frustration cause Qi to stagnate, which usually leads to constipation that is accompanied by abdominal distention. This results in a bloated sensation and sometimes physical pain.
- *Excess mental activity:* Working or thinking too much can make less Qi available for the transportation of food, which can ultimately lead to constipation. This kind, unlike the kind caused by emotional stress, is not accompanied by abdominal distention or pain.
- *Excess physical activity:* Too much physical labor or exercise can deplete Qi, resulting in overall dryness—including the dryness associated with constipation.
- *Lack of physical activity:* The right amount of labor or exercise stimulates Qi to do its proper job. Without this stimulation, stools move sluggishly and constipation occurs.
- *Repeated illness-related fevers:* Fevers generally use up fluid in the body, resulting in overall dryness, dry stools, and constipation.

Western Treatment

Dietary management (including foods high in fiber), mineral oil, laxatives, enemas, bowel training (geared toward having bowel movements at the same time each day), psychotherapy.

Chinese Treatment

For all kinds of constipation, do the following:

- Massage the abdomen in a clockwise motion.
- Rub the palms together in a circular motion (according to hand acupuncture, they correspond to the abdomen).
- Massage ST 25, and BL 25
- Massage the hand D micromeridian, which corresponds to the Large Intestine channel; this micromeridian is located on the back side and the back-hand side of the fourth finger, on the edge next to the fifth finger, from the tip to the hand.
- For children under age six:

  Massage the abdomen in a counterclockwise direction.

  Massage the lower vertebral column from L 4 (Lumbar 4, which corresponds to BL 25) to the tailbone (or coccyx) in a counterclockwise direction. In Chinese terms this area is called the Qiji ("seven knots or divisions") and Guiwei ("tail of the turtle"). This massage cleanses the body by making the elimination process work better.

- Increase intake of fruits and vegetables.
- Engage in a lifestyle that balances exercise, rest, work, and play.

Also do the following, depending upon which description best fits the situation:

- For cold constipation (infrequent stools, abdominal pain, pale face, feeling of general coldness or of cold hands and feet):

  Keep the navel (CV 8) warm, or put something warm over

it. A common Chinese remedy is to place a slice of heated ginger on top of the navel. This can be used for all ages, because ginger is a herb that transmits warmth through the navel into the abdomen.

Massage CV 6 to warm the Lower Burner; KI 6, BL 23 for general warmth; can also massage BL 25, and ST 25.

- For hot constipation (infrequent, dry stools; thirst; sometimes abdominal pain, red face, dry mouth): massage LI 11 to clear intestinal heat, TB 8 to clear heat and promote bowel movement, ST 44 to clear stomach heat, KI 3 and KI 6 to increase fluid, ST 25, and BL 25.
- For Qi deficiency (possible difficulty with bowel movement, infrequent but not very dry stools, easily tired, pale complexion): massage ST 36, SP 6, CV 6, KI 3, ST 25, and BL 25.

Cough

Symptoms

Sudden, noisy expulsion of air from the lungs through the mouth, possibly accompanied by dryness or tickling in the throat, phlegm, and/or tightness of the chest.

Description

Western medicine recognizes numerous possible causes of coughing, some of which have their own distinctive symptoms:

- *Common cold:* a viral or bacterial infection in the upper respiratory system. If viral, the cough may be accompanied by a low-grade fever and/or thin, clear, or white phlegm. If bacterial, the cough will be more severe and may be accompanied by thick, puslike, or yellow phlegm. For more information see *Cold, Common* in this guide.
- *Bronchitis:* a viral or viral-bacterial infection affecting one or both of the large airways (bronchi) leading to the lungs. The cough is deeper-sounding and rougher than a cough due to a common cold. The breath going through the airway

sounds like "rhonchi" through a stethoscope, indicating that the problem lies deeper in the chest than the upper respiratory system (associated with the common cold).

- *Pneumonia:* infection in lung tissue itself, possibly caused by viral or viral-bacterial infection, tuberculosis, parasites, or fungus. In this case, the examining doctor can detect (through a stethoscope) a thinner-breathing sound called "rales," which sounds like two pieces of sandpaper being rubbed together.

- *Asthma:* viral or bacterial infection in the smaller airways (bronchioles) of the respiratory system. Because air has to squeeze through narrower airways, there is a whistling sound called "wheezing." It can be heard with a stethoscope in milder cases, and even without one in more severe attacks. There is a general sensation of tightness in the chest. The cough usually sounds like a wheeze. For more information, see *Asthma* in this guide.

- *Other, less common causes:* aspiration, which occurs when a food particle accidentally gets in the airways; cancer; cystic fibrosis; emphysema; smoking; tuberculosis.

Like Western medicine, Chinese medicine attributes coughing to respiratory tract disorders but also takes into consideration problems in the person's overall diet, lifestyle, and living conditions, which can contribute to the duration, severity, or recurrence of a cough. Based on all these factors, Chinese medicine recognizes three major types of coughing conditions:

- *Wind Cold* (corresponds to viral infection): an acute, excess condition caused by external pathogens. It is the shortest-lasting, least problematic of the three major types. The pathogens most commonly enter the respiratory tract through the nose, mouth, and skin, where Defensive Qi circulates. They go on to disrupt the flow of Lung Qi, which naturally flows downward, as well as the functioning of the

Lung, which disperses Qi throughout the body. When this happens, Qi "rebels" upward, causing a cough.

Children are especially vulnerable to external pathogens due to their softer skin, which can more easily lead to weak Defensive Qi. Children are also more likely to go outside without sufficient clothing in the winter and spring, when temperature fluctuations are the most dramatic and, therefore, when external pathogens are more likely to cause trouble.

The symptoms that specifically point to a Wind Cold cough include thin, watery, white sputum; watery nasal discharge; an aversion to cold temperatures; low-grade or no fever; no sweating; and possibly muscle aches, headaches, or a sore throat.

- *Wind Heat* (corresponds to bacterial infection): a more serious condition caused in the same way as a Wind Cold condition (see above). The symptoms that specifically point to a Wind Heat condition are coughing with more effort or distress; sticky, yellow, thick sputum; thick nasal discharge; thirst, often accompanied by fever with some sweating; dry mouth; aversion to warm or hot temperatures; and possibly general malaise, generalized body aches, or headache.

  A related condition is Wind Dryness, which occurs when a person is exposed to sudden cold (e.g., air conditioning) after being in very warm weather (e.g., outdoors on a hot summer day). This situation induces a state of being hot inside and cold outside, which can produce a harsh, painful cough with a sore throat, sometimes accompanied by yellow phlegm and a feeling of chilliness.

- *Phlegm Damp:* This type of cough is caused by an internal weakness of the digestive system's Spleen. When the Spleen doesn't properly get rid of phlegm and dampness, it accumulates in the body, especially in the Lung and Spleen channels. In addition to causing a cough, this condition can prolong a cough caused by external factors (see "Wind Cold" and "Wind Heat" above).

Injury to the Lung and Spleen channels can be triggered by poor diet, stress, exposure to wetness (e.g., because of living in damp conditions), or overuse of antibiotics—all of which can deplete the body's Qi and possibly cause external pathogens to linger and do long-term damage. *Note:* Chinese experts believe that repeated or chronic use of antibiotics sometimes can lead to a vicious circle of recurrent coughing: antibiotic treatment for one cough-related illness results in weakened Lung and SP systems and therefore predisposess the body to another cough-related illness later, and so forth).

Also, when a person's Spleen Qi is weak, food is not properly digested. Instead, it ferments and becomes phlegm. This phlegm rises up into the lungs and obstructs them. Because they can no longer direct Qi downward, the Qi "rebels" upward, resulting in a cough.

Western Treatment

The most common treatment involves cough medications, either over-the-counter or prescription, of which there are two major types: expectorant (assists in coughing up phlegm) and suppressant (assists in reducing frequency and intensity of coughing). An antibiotic also may be prescribed, either to treat or to prevent a secondary infection, but in most cases this step is advisable only if there is good evidence of the possibility of a bacterial infection. Recommended home care includes lots of fluids, rest, and aspirin or some other antipyretic to reduce fever.

Chinese Treatment

Treatment for a cough is similar to that for a common cold (see *Cold, Common* in this guide). For all types of coughs, or for a Wind Cold cough in particular, do the following:
* Massage GB 20, the Wind Gate.

- Massage LI 4, LU 9, P 6, and CV 22.
- Massage ST 36 to strengthen the body's general immunity.
- Massage the upper back in a clockwise direction. Also massage BL 13.
- On the hand, tonify the C micromeridian and the corresponding points for the Lung and nose on the palm side of the third finger.
- Keep warm when there is any feeling of coldness or chills.
- Sweat to open the pores, which drives out pathogens and helps circulate Defensive Qi. This can be done by using a humidifier, sitting in a steamed bathroom, or lowering the towel-draped head over a sink or basin of hot water.
- Drink lots of fluids. (For a Wind Cold cough, chicken soup would be nourishing.)
- Decrease ingestion of or avoid cold foods and drinks.

For a Wind Heat cough, add the following treatments:
- Massage DU 14 to alleviate fever.
- Massage LI 11.
- Massage LU 10 counterclockwise and LU 5 clockwise to clear heat from the lungs.
- Reduce intake of heat-producing foods, such as garlic or onions. Chicken soup in some instances may be too warm for the Wind Heat cough.

For a Phlegm Damp cough, add the following treatments to the general ones listed above:
- Massage the upper and the middle back clockwise.
- Massage ST 40, SP 6, LU 9, and ST 36.
- Apply heated ginger to the navel.
- Reduce ingestion of or avoid phlegm-producing foods (e.g., bananas, cow's milk or cheese, peanut butter, peanuts, and sugar).
- Reduce stress and workload.

- Do the following, as appropriate:

  To alleviate body aches, massage LR 3.

  To calm the person (e.g., children can be easily agitated by a fever), massage HT 7.

  To alleviate nausea and vomiting, massage P 6.

Consult a physician in the event of a lingering cough that is unresponsive to medication; a serious cough suggestive of bronchitis, pneumonia, or asthma (see symptoms noted above under "Description"); or a cough that brings up blood or phlegm containing blood.

Diaper Rash

Symptoms

In the diaper area, red patches with "satellite" lesions—small red dots surrounding the rash itself.

Description

Western medicine attributes diaper rash to a yeast overgrowth in moist areas, which sometimes can be accompanied by a secondary bacterial infection. *Note:* Antibiotic therapy for some other illness can alter the normal state of yeast or bacteria in the diaper area and trigger or complicate a case of diaper rash.

Chinese medicine associates diaper rash with a damp heat condition (see *Eczema* in this guide for a fuller explanation).

Western Treatment

Antiyeast cream such as Nystatin Cream; steroid hydrocortisone cream for inflammation and itchiness; antibacterial cream when there is secondary bacterial infection with pus drainage. Also, keep the diaper area dry, change diapers frequently, and if possible leave the baby without a diaper for a time.

Chinese Treatment

Massage LU 5, LI 4, LI 11, LR 3, LR 8, ST 40, and SP 10. Also, avoid foods that produce excess phlegm or heat. In addition, follow the same Western treatment recommendations listed above regarding diapers.

Diarrhea

Symptoms

Loose or watery stools and usually increased frequency of defecation, possibly accompanied by abdominal pain and fever.

Description

Diarrhea can be divided into two categories: acute and chronic. Each category is discussed individually below.

1. *Acute diarrhea:* In both Western and Chinese medicine, the major concern with acute diarrhea is dehydration or fluid loss. This issue is especially critical in the case of young children, who can become dehydrated very quickly.

Signs of mild-to-moderate dehydration include dry lips, lack of tears, and sunken eyes; also, in infants, listlessness and a sunken fontanelle (a soft spot located on the top of the head toward the front; it is a normal finding in babies up to 1 year of age).

Signs of moderate-to-severe dehydration include doughy-feeling skin, pale complexion, cold limbs, and decreased urination. This latter degree of dehydration may require emergency care (intravenous fluid administration).

In Western terms, acute diarrhea can be caused by viral, bacterial, or parasitic infection; or by food poisoning, which is triggered by toxins released from contaminated bacteria in the food.

Chinese medicine features a broader point of view on diarrhea that incorporates the Western explanations under categories relating to cold, dampness, and heat in the following ways:

Cold-damp invasion: This category includes the Western diagnoses of viral infections and food poisoning but also involves cases that are caused strictly by coldness and dampness. Either way, coldness and dampness accumulate in the Stomach and Intestines, resulting in an obstruction of Qi and, accordingly, diarrhea. Specific symptoms include watery, slightly foul-smelling stools; abdominal pain; loss of appetite; borborygmi (stomach growlings); myalgia (muscle aches); general malaise; headache; and an aversion to cold.

Heat-damp invasion: This category includes the Western diagnoses of bacterial infections but also involves cases that are caused strictly by heat (especially summer heat) and dampness. The heat and dampness enter the Large Intestine and impede Qi flow. Specific symptoms include the symptoms for cold-damp invasion (except for an aversion to cold) along with fever (or a feeling of warmth) and a burning sensation in the rectum and the anus.

2. *Chronic diarrhea:* In Western terms, chronic diarrhea results from any of the following conditions: a damaged intestinal wall due to recurrent, protracted diarrhea; chronic anatomical or biochemical abnormalities (such as inflammatory bowel disease, malabsorption syndrome, or enzyme/hormone deficiencies); congenital abnormalities (such as lactose intolerance); or recurrent infections.

   In Chinese terms, chronic diarrhea, like any other chronic illness, is related to a Qi disturbance caused by improper diet, emotional stress, and/or an unbalanced lifestyle, such as one that involves working too hard. Both the Digestive Qi and the KI Yang aspects of the body are affected as follows:

Digestive Qi deficiency: In a typical case of chronic diarrhea, the person has diarrhea two to three times a day, occasionally with undigested food particles, as well as abdominal pain and distention. The pain and distention may be relieved by a foul-smelling bowel movement, often occurring immediately or soon after eating. Other symptoms include poor appetite, fatigue, sallow (yellowish) complexion, and general paleness. In some cases the person's eyes remain only half closed during sleep. If mild dehydration sets in, the urine is scanty and concentrated.

A Digestive Qi weakness may be hereditary, which, in Western terms, corresponds to a genetic malabsorption syndrome or an enzyme deficiency. Improper diet factors include an excess of cold foods, drugs (such as antibiotics), milk (which contributes to Qi-injuring dampness), and greasy or sweet foods. Excessive thinking and worrying also harm Digestive Qi.

KI Yang deficiency: Kidney Yang is the foundation of all Yang energy in the body and correlates to genetic predisposition in Western medicine. A KI Yang deficiency may be congenital or it may result from prolonged diarrhea, which leads to coldness in the entire digestive system. The symptoms include early morning diarrhea, abdominal pain, and intolerance to cold.

Western Treatment

For acute diarrhea: the first order of treatment is to resupply the body with water (rehydration). Initially restrict the fluid intake to small amounts of clear liquids, consumed frequently (such as every half hour). Gradually advance the diet to include other liquids, then semisolids, as tolerated, always watching for signs of dehydration. Antidiarrheal medications, both prescription and over-the-counter, can be taken for a short period (typically up to two days) to alleviate especially severe attacks. Severe diarrhea with dehydration may require IV therapy.

For chronic diarrhea: dehydration is not as important to address as it is for acute attacks. Instead, the case needs medical evaluation to determine specific causes and treatments.

Chinese Treatment

For acute diarrhea: follow the same fluid and dietary guidelines given under "Western Treatment" above, with these additions:

For invasion by Cold-Damp, also do the following:
- Massage the Middle Burner on the back in clockwise fashion or apply gentle heat to that area.
- Massage the abdomen in a counterclockwise direction.
- Massage CV 12, SP 6, SP 9, CV 6, ST 25, and ST 40.
- Massage the fingers: the D micromeridian on the back of the fourth finger, on the side closest to the fifth finger; massage from the hand to the fingertip.
- Massage the F micromeridian on the middle of the palm side of the fifth finger, from the tip toward the palm.
- Apply a slice of heated ginger on the navel (CV 8).

For children under age six:
- Massage the lower vertebral column from L 4 to the coccyx (tailbone) in a counterclockwise direction. In Chinese terms this area is called the Qiji ("seven knots or divisions") and Guiwei ("tail of the turtle"). This massage cleanses the body by making the elimination process work better.

For invasion by Heat-Damp, also do the following:
- the treatments for invasion by Cold-Damp listed above
- Massage LI 4 and LI 11 to expel heat from the Large Intestine.

For chronic diarrhea: In addition to the treatments for acute diarrhea, invasion by Cold-Damp listed above, do the following:

For Digestive Qi deficiency:
- Massage P 6 if vomiting occurs.
- Massage SP 4 to alleviate abdominal distention.
- Alter your diet or lifestyle to avoid excesses that are cited above as possible causes.

For KI Yang deficiency:
- Massage DU 4 and BL 23 to warm the Kidney Mingmen (Life Gate) area in the lower back.
- Massage the Lower Burner in a clockwise direction.
- Massage KI 3 and KI 7.
- On the hand, massage the J micromeridian channel on the back-hand side of the fifth finger, from the tip toward the palm.

Drooling

Symptoms

Excess secretion of saliva from the mouth.

Description

Drooling occurs when there is less swallowing or closing of the lips or when there is an irritation in the mouth, such as when infants teethe. It also can be a reflex response when anticipating feeding or pain. In addition, people suffering from a central nervous system disorder such as a stroke or from mental retardation frequently have excessive drooling.

Chinese medicine further attributes drooling to a Wind insult to the face, which weakens the facial muscles for swallowing, or to excess heat in the mouth (caused by previous infections), which stimulates more saliva for cooling. Other causes may be a diet heavy in phlegm-producing foods, which results in an overall increase in body fluids; a weakness in the Digestive Qi system; and a weakness in the KI regulation of fluid.

Western Treatment

Usually medications, which can result in overdryness and dental decay; in extreme cases, removal of salivary glands.

Chinese Treatment

To properly treat the drooling, consult a professional to determine the underlying cause. To alleviate it, do the following:
• Massage ST 4, SI 1, KI 7.

Ear Infection

Symptoms

Ear pain, possibly accompanied by discharge from the ear canal, redness in or warmness of the external ear, fluid or redness behind the eardrum (seen with an otoscope), and/or fever (especially in children).

Description

Western medicine distinguishes two categories of infection within the ear canal: outside the eardrum (otitis externa or OE), or inside the eardrum (otitis media or OM).

OEs usually are acute in nature—that is, they come on suddenly and last for a short period of time. The most common causes are a cold or an aftereffect of swimming ("swimmer's ear"). OMs are classified as either acute (AOM) or as chronic serous (CSOM; serous means fluid-producing). AOM is due to fluid buildup in the middle ear, which has become secondarily infected. Even after each acute infection has cleared, the fluid still stays in the middle ear, so that recurrent or persistent AOM frequently results in the more problematic CSOM.

AOM is most prevalent among children of age eight months to two years. Half of these children will have recurrences of AOM into their early elementary school years. The most common causes of AOM are allergies or bacterial or viral infections.

Chinese medicine doesn't classify ear infection as either OE or OM, but it does distinguish between acute and chronic otitis. Acute otitis is due to the invasion of an external pathogen, resulting in a coldness that slows down Qi and blood movement; fluid accumulation that fosters bacterial infection; and heat accumulation in the ear and head. Chronic otitis is caused by a more general Qi or Yin imbalance.

Western Treatment

Generally, OE is treated with ear drops: antibiotics or steroids. AOM may be treated with ear drops for pain as well as oral decongestants, analgesics, and antibiotics. CSOM is often treated with maintenance antibiotic therapy consisting of a daily dose of antibiotics for several months to prevent recurrence of the infection.

Chinese Treatment

For acute otitis, do the following:
- Massage LI 4, ST 36, and ST 44 to disperse heat from the head.
- Massage GB 20.
- Massage the ear points TB 21, SI 19, and GB 2 to bring healing energy to the ear.
- Massage DU 14 to alleviate fever.
- Massage the sides of the topmost segment of the third finger on the palm side—these correspond to mapping of the ears onto the hands.
- Avoid phlegm-producing foods and excessive intake of cold foods.

For chronic otitis (including recurring cases of acute otitis within a relatively short period of time), massage ST 36. Also do the following, depending on which description better fits the situation:

For chronic otitis, considered to be a Yin deficiency, associated with lower back and knee soreness, fatigue, pale face with flushed cheeks, night sweat, and/or dry mouth:
- Massage KI 3 and KI 6.
- Massage TB 21, SI 19, and GB 2—the ear points
- Massage the lower back in a clockwise direction to strengthen Kidney Qi.

- Massage the J micromeridian on the back and outside of the fifth finger—massage from the tip toward the hand.

For recurrent acute otitis, considered to be a Spleen deficiency associated with sallow (yellowish) complexion, decreased appetite, and/or fatigue:

- Massage SP 3 and SP 6.
- Massage the midback in a clockwise direction to strengthen the digestive system.
- Massage the F micromeridian: the middle of the fifth finger on the palm side, massage from the tip toward the palm.

Ear-Ringing (Tinnitus)

Symptoms

Hearing noise in one or both ears; may be a ringing, buzzing, whistling, hissing, roaring, high-pitched sound, or rushing-water sound, or a bell-like tone; may be accompanied by some degree of deafness.

Description

Ear-ringing is very common among adults. From the standpoint of Western medicine, it may indicate a relatively insignificant problem, such as wax blocking the eustachian tube (ear canal). Alternatively, it may be due to a variety of causes, including flu, ear infection, perforation of the eardrum, hypertension, or a tumor in the cranium.

Ear-ringing in one ear (unilateral tinnitus) with a bell-like tone and reduced hearing generally suggests a disease within the ear. Sounds like rushing water or escaping steam indicate a disease of the auditory nerve. Hearing one's pulse in the ear may simply be a sign that the person is very introspective (i.e., predisposed to be inward and therefore more receptive to interior body noises), or it could indicate intracranical vascular malformation (malformation of blood vessels in the brain). Medications such as aspirin and other salicylates or quinine also can trigger temporary ear-ringing or deafness. Other causes include foreign infectious agents and exposure to loud sounds (such as listening to loud music with headphones).

Chinese medicine attributes ear-ringing to a Qi disturbance caused by any of the following:

- *Dietary problems:* These include excess intake of phlegm-producing foods that prevent clear Qi from rising to the head.
- *Emotional upset:* Prolonged anger, irritability, frustration, depression, worry, or grief can weaken different Qi systems so that ear-ringing takes place whenever another strong episode of the emotion occurs.
- *Adverse lifestyle habits:* Working too hard, excessive sexual activity, and old age wear down the Kidney, the foundation of the body's Qi and Essence and which is linked to the ear. A symptom of this cause may be a low-pitched sound in the ear.

Over a period of time, any of the above causes can undermine the health of one's organs and meridians, resulting in an imbalance in one's Qi or blood—a situation that also could account for many of the Western medical diagnoses listed above. The imbalance may be characterized as either an excessive or a deficient condition.

To help determine if the condition is excessive or deficient, cover the ears with the hands; if the ringing gets worse, the condition is probably excessive. One type of excessive condition is caused by an external disease-causing agent. If so, the illness generally features a sudden onset of ear-ringing accompanied by fever and headache. This correlates with the Western diagnosis of acute infection. Another type of excessive condition, caused by an excess of Liver and Gallbladder Qi, is directly related to an upsetting emotional experience, especially one featuring anger or depression. Possible symptoms of this type, in addition to ear-ringing, are a dry throat and a bitter taste in the mouth.

A deficient condition is usually indicated by a lessening of the ear-ringing problem when the ears are covered. It is often accompanied by deafness, knee or back pain, blurred vision, and/or dizziness.

Western Treatment

Based on professional testing. A careful history is taken to eliminate possible causes such as medication use/abuse or prolonged exposure to loud noises (e.g., listening to music set at a high volume). In rare cases, an angiogram is performed to rule out blood vessel malformation.

Chinese Treatment

For either an excessive or a deficient condition, massage the following points:

- The ear points TB 21, SI 19, and GB 2; also can add TB 5, GB 20, and LI 4.
- For an excessive condition, add LR 3 and GB 40.
- For a deficient condition, add KI 3, CV 4, CV 6, and the middle and lower back together, in a clockwise direction.

Eczema

Symptoms

When acute: redness and weepy, small blisters; when chronic: dry, scaly, thickened skin with darker-color change.

Description

In terms of Western medicine, eczema is an allergic skin condition that may be due to direct skin contact with an allergen or to the manifestation of allergens that have gotten into the body via the respiratory or digestive tract. It frequently occurs in asthmatics who react to various allergens.

As perceived by Chinese medicine, the skin, which breathes, is an extension of the Lungs and circulates Defensive Qi. The

197

skin is highly vulnerable to Lung disorders, which helps explain why asthmatics frequently have eczema. In addition, the skin is sensitive to dampness and heat accumulations, an excess condition that can result in an acute case of eczema lesions. A chronic case of eczema is a sign of a deficiency condition that has affected the blood, causing the skin to turn dry and scaly because of insufficient blood nourishment.

Western Treatment

Steroid creams; also avoidance of things that tend to cause an allergic reaction.

Chinese Treatment

For an acute case of eczema, massage LU 5, LI 11, ST 40, and SP 10. Also, avoid foods that produce excess phlegm.

For a chronic case of eczema, follow the guidelines for an acute case and add the following massages:

- BL 17, the back Shu point that tonifies the blood, located in the middle of the back in an area level with the lower border of the shoulder blade
- the hand meridian F that corresponds to the Spleen channel, located in the middle of the palm side of the fifth finger; massage from the tip to the palm

Edema (Swelling)

Symptoms

Swelling of body tissues, cavities, or organs.

Description

Edema occurs when there is excess fluid in body tissues, cavities, or organs. It does not occur in bones. The fluid can be one or more of various types: blood, lymph (carries fluids to the bloodstream, cleans toxic substances from it, and fights disease); synovial fluid (lubricates joints); serous fluid; and urine.

According to Western medicine, there are many possible causes of edema, including any condition that involves failure of the heart, kidney, or liver (causing excess fluid accumulation); low blood protein (causing the spread of blood and fluid beyond the vessel wall); and localized obstructions (e.g., a tumor in the leg that impedes fluid movement).

Chinese medicine maintains that body fluids, originating from food and drink, go through an intricate series of purification processes. First they are transformed and separated by the Spleen. The "clean" part of these fluids goes up to the Lungs, which send a portion to the Skin and a portion to the Kidneys. A "dirty" part goes down to the Small Intestine, where it is further separated into "pure" and "impure" parts. The pure part goes to the Large Intestine, which reabsorbs a portion of it as water. The impure part goes to the Bladder, which further transforms it into a pure part that flows upward and becomes sweat, and an impure part that flows downward and becomes urine.

To summarize this process as a whole, clean/pure fluids go upward, while dirty/impure fluids go downward. The Spleen functions as the "prime mover." To use a Western analogy, the Spleen is like a large lymph node filtering out toxins and distributing beneficial liquids. Therefore the Spleen is always treated in Chinese medicine whenever there is any disorder involving body fluids. Other important organs to treat are the Lungs, Kidney, and Stomach.

Western Treatment

Doctors decrease fluid volume with diuretics, then treat the underlying cause or causes—for example, by prescribing heart medications for congestive heart failure.

Chinese Treatment

For edema anywhere on the body, massage the following points or areas:

199

- SP 6, SP 9, BL 20, BL 22, BL 23, KI 7, and ST 43
- the midback and the lower back, each in a circular, clockwise motion
- KI 6, KI 7, CV 3, CV 5, and CV 7 or, alternatively, the midline of the abdomen, from the pubic area toward the navel
- CV 9 and LU 5

For edema of the four limbs, also massage KI 7, GB 43, and SP 2.

For edema of the lower limbs, also massage KI 7 and LU 5.

For edema in the abdomen, also massage CV 9.

Emotional Problems

Symptoms

Emotional problems are complex in nature and difficult to label precisely, but the most often cited emotions relating to the Five Elements are sadness/grief, fear, joy/passion, anxiety/frustration/anger, and worry.

A person's emotional difficulties may involve a combination of these emotions as well as others—a fact that's not always apparent on the surface. For this reason it is important to review the entire entry and gain a broad perspective on emotional problems and their treatments, rather than to focus only on information relating to a particular emotion.

For other symptoms relating to Chinese medical categories, see "Description" below.

Description

From a Western medical perspective, emotional problems are caused by a complex assortment of factors, including any combination of the following: poor physical health; biochemical irregularities; psychological predispositions; environmental, social, or situational impacts; poor diet; and/or substance abuse.

According to Chinese medicine, Mind (which includes emotions or inner feelings) and Body are intimately connected. Another part of a human being that is closely integrated with Mind and Body is Spirit. In fact, the Chinese word *Shen* is translated as both Mind and Spirit. The spiritual part of a human being refers to how he or she relates to the world outside of oneself—the immediate circle of family, friends, associates, work, recreation; the larger realm of community, state, country; and ultimately Nature, the Universe. A problem in any of these three aspects of the being may resonate in the other two; For example, problematic physical symptoms often result in a Qi imbalance that influences the emotional equilibrium, which, in turn, may eventually upset the spiritual balance.

Treatment involves establishing which Yin organs in the body are most involved in the problem. Each Yin organ is associated with a particular emotional and spiritual area, as follows:

Yin Organ and Emotional and Spiritual Aspects

Yin Organ	Emotion(s)	Spiritual Aspect(s)
Kidney	fear	willpower
Liver	anger, irritability, frustration, hatred	Ethereal Soul: connection to the "universal" spirit
Heart	joy, passion, love, desire, guilt	Mind—all-encompassing
Spleen/Pancreas	sympathy, compassion, worry	intelligence
Lung	sadness, grief	Corporeal Soul: defines physical being/senses

Each of these organ-based categories is discussed more specifically below. When figuring out the nature of any emotional problem, it's important to review all the categories to determine possible areas of relevance.

Kidney: fear and long-term grief without tears

- Fear in this category relates specifically to a new situation, change, or some sort of phobia, as opposed to fear relating to decisionmaking (which falls in the Liver category).
- Over the years, grief that is tolerated without tears (in other words, which goes unexpressed) upsets the fluid mechanism within the Kidneys.
- Physical symptoms include becoming easily tired, feeling weak, paleness, dizziness, poor hearing, and/or backache.
- Mental/emotional/spiritual symptoms include a lack of will-power, motivation, and drive (as opposed to a lack of direction—a Liver-related problem), and/or poor memory for life-related events (as opposed to poor memory for facts—a Spleen-related problem).

Liver: anger, frustration, irritability, hatred

- Other Liver-related emotional problems include resentment, rage, indignation, or bitterness.
- There are two major combinations of physical and mental/emotional/spiritual symptoms, as follows:
  1. Physical symptoms include mild dizziness, numbness of the limbs, inability to fall asleep, blurred vision, scanty or no menstrual flow, dull to pale complexion, muscle cramps, and/or brittle nails.

     Mental/emotional/spiritual symptoms include lacking a sense of direction and vision in life, confusion about goals, and/or fear of making wrong decisions.
  2. Physical symptoms include thirst, a bitter taste, dizziness, ear-ringing, dream-disturbed sleep, a floating sensation immediately before falling asleep, headache, red face and eyes, dark urine, and/or dry stools.

     Mental/emotional/spiritual symptoms include irritability, frustration, impulsiveness, and/or underlying anger that may not be expressed or that may manifest as depres-

sion; expressed anger may take the form of shouting at people or physical aggressiveness.
- Anger can easily spread from the Liver to affect other areas, such as the Heart, the Digestive System, and the Kidney. The counterpart of anger is dynamic power, creativity, and generosity. This means that the same energy dissipated in outbursts of anger can be harnessed to help a person achieve more positive life goals.

Heart: joy, passion, love (in an excess state, obsessive passion)
- All emotions eventually affect the Heart, known as the "Emperor Organ." It is the residence for Shen (Mind and Spirit).
- In its optimum state, the Heart is relaxed, calm, and able to focus. An excess state results in too much stimulation, craving, jealousy, or obsessive passion (as opposed to Spleen-based obsession with everyday life events).
- Physical symptoms include palpitations, inability to fall asleep or frequent waking during the night, fidgetiness, talking a lot, mild dizziness, dull to pale complexion, being easily startled, and/or tiredness.
- Mental/emotional/spiritual symptoms include mild, free-floating anxiety; sense of unease, especially in the evening; overexcitability; poor memory; depression; a tendency toward aggressiveness; and/or any or all of three major types of mental states: mind obstructed: thinking unclear, loss of insight; mind restless or agitated and anxious; and mind weakened— mentally tired and depressed.

Spleen/Pancreas: sympathy, compassion, worry
- The Spleen/Pancreas controls thinking and intellectual functioning relating to data and tasks (e.g., at school or at work). When it's balanced, a person can concentrate, memorize facts, and learn.

- It also governs sympathy and compassion (as opposed to passion) relating to others. When it's balanced, a person is appropriately caring and nurturing.
- Physical symptoms include digestive problems, such as poor appetite; dry mouth; slight throat pain; sallow complexion; and/or feeling of heaviness in the body.
- Mental/emotional/spiritual symptoms include the following:
  1. poor memory and concentration/inattentiveness for work, learning, tests; dull thoughts; mental confusion; in severe cases, may lead to obsession or inability to think
- 2. subdued state of mind, quietness, excessive concern or excessive worry about people or things; in severe cases, obsessive worry about someone or something (as opposed to pathological obsessive passion that relates to the Heart)

Lung: sadness, grief, depression
- The Lung is associated with grief that is expressed in tears and weepy depression.
- The Lung is responsible for deriving Qi from the air and directing it to other parts of the body. When Lung Qi is weak, the person is adversely affected in all ways, including emotionally. The opposite is true as well: when a person is mentally, emotionally, and spiritually unbalanced, Lung Qi is negatively affected.
- Physical symptoms include quickness to cry, paleness, fatigue, slower physical movements, breathlessness, pressing sensation on the chest, dry throat, and/or nonspecific physical discomfort (e.g., itchy skin).
- Mental/emotional/spiritual symptoms include being easily influenced by emotional stimuli; loneliness; sadness; being subdued; and speaking in a lower, softer voice.

Individual vulnerability to a particular emotion depends on the following factors:
- *Physical constitution:* This includes genetic makeup, such as an

inherited weakness in an organ or predisposition to a certain kind of emotional illness; also includes any events during the prenatal period, such as a mother's drug addiction, weakening the Liver Qi transmitted to the unborn infant.

- *Family influence:* Many emotional problems have their onset in childhood, based on interactions with parents and siblings. Among the possible negative influences are lack of demonstrated affection from a parent; an upbringing that is overly lenient or overly strict; a parent's alcoholism; sibling rivalry; fighting between parents or siblings; a parent's excessive or inappropriate expectations; residual feelings following a death or a divorce in the family; a parent's overdependence on a child (e.g., as the result of a death or divorce in the family).

- *Diet:* Different kinds of foods and drugs affect different Qi channels and organs; for example, excessive alcohol consumption creates a hotness that causes injury to the Liver and the Heart.

- *Lifestyle:* Excessive indulgence in any activity—physical exercise, work, sex, studying—causes an imbalance of Qi flow, which leads to an imbalance of body systems.

Western Treatment

If you suspect a serious emotional problem, it is best to consult a professional, as emotional problems are usually complex in nature and difficult to define or treat on one's own. Individual cases are diagnosed by professionals as being either acute (a short-term condition based on a recent event, such as the death of a family member) or chronic (a long-term condition, such as unresolved grief from a death many years ago).

Often the treatment is the same for either an acute or a chronic situation: medication for relaxation, psychotropic medications (those that alter mental functioning, such as antidepressant drugs), and/or some form of psychotherapy based on individual preference and the nature of the problem (such as

Freudian, Jungian, transpersonal, Gestalt, family-based, or other forms of therapy). Drugs usually treat only the symptoms of the problem, not the root cause or causes. Psychotherapy aims to do the latter.

Chinese Treatment

Chinese medical experts, like Western medical experts, recommend consultation with a professional if a serious emotional problem is suspected. However, there are certain steps, recommended below, that can be taken at home to help alleviate the problem. Ideally they would be taken in conjunction with a more specifically targeted, professionally administered program of acupuncture, which, in addition to providing a better end result, would increase the effectiveness of the healing work done at home. Here are steps for dealing with an emotional problem at home:

1. Review the information provided in this entry to determine as best you can the general type of imbalance or imbalances that exist: that is, the organ or organs, Qi type or types, and channel or channels involved. There may be more than one type of imbalance.
2. Based on your determination, follow any appropriate dietary and meditation suggestions given in this book.
3. Working with three different areas of the back—upper, middle, and lower—massage the points below that are most appropriate to the problem:

Upper Back

BL 42: Window of the Corporeal Soul, next to the Lung Shu point
- treats Lung type of sadness and grief
- frees any heavy sensation of the chest associated with depression and worry
- relieves nonspecific physical sensations such as itchiness

- makes the person feel more comfortable within his or her body

BL 44: Shen Palace, next to Heart Shu point
- calms the Mind
- clears thinking and stimulates memory
- relieves Mind of obsessive passion

Middle Back

BL 47: Hunmen, Door of the Ethereal Soul, next to the Liver Shu point (*Note:* The Ethereal Soul resides in the Liver Yin.)
- strengthens and roots the Ethereal Soul so that the Mind functions better
- increases one's ability to plan, to have a better sense of purpose and direction, and to carry ideas to completion
- helps overcome depression associated with Liver imbalance

BL 49: Yishe, the Hut of the Intellect, next to the Spleen Shu point
- strengthens intellect
- improves learning and memory for data and tasks
- enhances concentration for school and for work
- relieves the mind of obsessive thoughts about life events
Note: It is advisable to massage the upper and middle back points (above) with the lower back point for the Kidney and willpower (below) so the Ethereal Soul is not overly stimulated without being grounded.

Lower Back

BL 52: Zhishi, Room of the Willpower, next to Kidney Shu points
- strengthens motivation, will power, drive, and the ability to set and achieve goals
- helps overcome fear

4. Massage the acupressure points below that are appropriate for the problem:

HT 7: calms the Mind and nourishes the Heart; alleviates physical symptoms related to Heart disturbance, such as palpitations

P 6: calms the Mind and improves the mood; opens the chest, which is good for physical feelings of tightness or oppressiveness in the chest; good for any emotional upset of the Heart, such as passion from the breakup of a relationship

Note: Massaging SP 4 along with P 6 can further relax the chest and calm the mind.

LR 3: helps alleviate repressed anger

DU 20: clears the Mind; improves thinking, concentration, and memory; relieves depression

ST 40: calms and clears the Mind

KI 3: helps alleviate Kidney-related symptoms and fear

GB 40: helps increase the ability to make decisions

LU 7: has a releasing effect on sadness, worry, and grief; helps alleviate the feeling of tightness in the chest

CV 15: good for calming the Mind and alleviating a feeling of tightness in the chest; helps relieve anxiety, insomnia, and mental restlessness

CV 17 and CV 6: increases feeling of energy; uplifts the spirit

Fatigue

Symptoms

A feeling of exhaustion after exertion of the body (physical fatigue) or mind (mental/emotional fatigue).

Description

Everyone feels fatigued or tired some of the time—this is most often a normal consequence of working, playing, or living too hard, or of undergoing significant mental or emotional strain. In some cases fatigue can be associated with a chronic physical or mental-emotional illness, what Westerners know as lung or heart disease, diabetes, hypothyroidism, cancer, depression, anemia, etc.

Chronic fatigue syndrome is a debilitating condition occurring over the course of months or even years. The cause is still unknown to Western medicine, but it's often associated with viral infections, especially the Epstein-Barr virus.

Chinese medicine also relates fatigue to chronic illness. It often results from excess conditions that impede the circulation of Qi and blood. The Liver is the most vulnerable organ for these conditions. Another source of fatigue is a deficiency illness in any major organ or meridian, which can result in insufficient Qi. Other fatigue-causing factors include restrictive or specialized diets, a diet too heavy in one kind of food (e.g., cold foods), mental or physical overexertion, too much sexual activity, and the use of certain drugs, such as marijuana.

Western Treatment

Specific professional treatment is directed at the underlying cause of fatigue. For home treatment of normal fatigue, rest and beneficial changes in lifestyle (such as decreasing the workload or eating more sensibly) are advised.

Chinese Treatment

Just as in Western medicine, specific professional treatment is designed to fit the particular condition or conditions underlying the fatigue. However, massaging the following points helps tonify the body and increase short-term energy regardless of the underlying cause of fatigue:

- ST 36. Called the "Walk Three Mile" point, ST 36 was discovered in ancient times by weary foot soldiers massaging their tired legs. They noticed that this one point was always the most sore or tender, so they massaged it more, and as a result got a surge of new energy—enough to walk another three miles. Ancient textbooks refer to this point as the "Cure Everything" point. In modern times it has come to be known as the "Master Immunity Point" because of its effectiveness in strengthening the immune system.

- CV 6: the "Sea of Qi" point
- KI 3
- DU 4
- DU 20

In addition to massaging these points, it is advisable to make sure one's diet and lifestyle are well balanced.

Gastritis
(also see *Abdominal Pain* and *Nervous Stomach*)

Symptoms

The most common symptoms are stomachache, pain in the esophagus or epigastric (throat) area, and loss of appetite, possibly accompanied by a sense of nausea and weight loss. Other symptoms are listed under "Description" below.

Description

Western medicine defines gastritis as an inflammation of the stomach lining. There also may be a break or breaks in the lining (erosion) causing bleeding (hemorrhage). The condition may be chronic, with either scarring and thickening, or thinning of the stomach lining. A chronic condition predisposes the stomach lining to develop ulcers.

There are multiple possible causes of erosive and hemorrhagic gastritis, including alcoholism, excessive intake of certain medications (such as aspirin), some chemotherapies, another serious illness accompanied by stress, trauma, or bacterial or viral infections, and parasites. Psychological stress also may be involved in the development of any kind of gastritis. Some cases (called idiopathic) have no identifiable cause.

In Chinese medicine, gastritis is considered an excess condition that has progressed from Heat in the Stomach to the more advanced and severe condition of Stomach Fire.

The causes of this condition include excess hot foods; infection; emotional turmoil, especially expressed anger, which can strongly affect the Stomach; excess mental work; eating irregularly over a long period of time (usually several years), which can cause a Stomach Yin deficiency and a corresponding increase in heat; and medications that can cause gastrointestinal symptoms.

Possible accompanying symptoms include thirst, irritability, dry mouth, red face, constipation, vomiting of blood from the stomach, and/or bleeding gums.

Western Treatment

Consult a physician for specific treatment: decrease ingestion of aggravating medications or foods; treat for infections; and seek counseling and possibly psychotherapy for stress and alcoholism.

Chinese Treatment

Do the following things, as appropriate:

Massage these points:
- ST 44, LI 11 to clear Stomach heat
- BL 21 or, alternatively, the midback in a clockwise motion
- ST 45; especially when epigastric pain is accompanied by excess irritability
- SP 6
- CV 12

Eat more regularly, decreasing the intake of hot foods and alcohol.
Decrease the amount of mental exertion in your life.
Avoid excess expression of anger.

211

Headache

Symptoms

Sharp or dull pain in the head, in one location or generalized; may be accompanied by unusual visual images (known as "visual aura"), such as seeing stars or spots in front of the eyes; nausea; or vomiting.

Description

In Western medicine, the two most common headaches are classified as tension-type (about 75% of adult headaches) and migraine (about 15–20%). There are a variety of possible causes for these and other types of headaches, including muscle contraction (especially for tension-type headaches), viral infection (e.g., a headache associated with a cold or a more serious condition such as meningitis), emotional stress, heredity (especially for migraine headaches), allergies (e.g., sinus headaches), a brain tumor, high blood pressure, or head trauma (a blow to the head causing a blood clot in the brain covering).

Because a headache can be a symptom of a serious physical illness, it's wise to consult a doctor if the pain is unusually severe, lingering, or incapacitating, or if it occurs early in the morning or is accompanied by other symptoms such as vomiting, fever, or stiffness of the neck.

Chinese medicine classifies headaches as either acute or chronic, or recurrent, as follows:

1. *Acute:* Isolated, sudden-onset headaches are mostly attributed to wind invasion. Wind by itself can enter into the body's channels to cause headaches (and possibly stiffness of the neck), or it can carry infectious agents along with it. Dampness also can trigger headaches, usually accompanied by a feeling of heaviness.

2. *Chronic, recurrent:* Headaches of this nature, like all other chronic, recurrent illnesses, usually are linked with problems

relating to one's diet, emotions, or lifestyle (an exception would be a chronic, recurrent headache caused by head trauma). Each of these factors is discussed as follows:

- *Diet:* Not eating enough or following a diet that is very restrictive and therefore not nutritionally sound causes a deficiency of Qi, resulting in headaches on the top of the head.

  Overeating causes headaches on the forehead that often feature sharp pain. Excess intake of hot foods or alcohol can generate sharp headaches on the front or sides of the head. Excess intake of greasy foods, dairy products, or sweets can cause dull, achy frontal headaches or a general sensation of heaviness in the head. Excess consumption of salt or sour foods also can lead to headaches. Salt-generated ones are dull and achy and may manifest themselves as headaches in the eye region ("frontal headaches").

  One's manner of eating also may be responsible. Eating too fast or with too much distraction (such as eating while working or watching TV) can lead to sharp frontal headaches. Another cause may be chemicals in one's food, such as caffeine or monosodium glutamate.

- *Emotions:* Strong, troublesome emotions, especially anger, frequently cause headaches. Emotional distress leads to Qi disturbance (usually stagnation) and fire rising to the head. The Western concept of being "hot-tempered," for example, corresponds to the Chinese medical concept that an angry person has an excess of fire in the head.

  From the perspective of Chinese medicine, what are called migraine headaches in Western medicine are often caused by emotional stress. For many women, ongoing emotional stress usually results in headaches before or during menstruation.

  Anger-related headaches tend to be felt on the sides or temples of the head. Worry-related headaches are usually dull and on the top of the head. Headaches resulting from an emotional shock are usually felt throughout the head.

- *Lifestyle:* Excess work that involves numerous mental activities or eyestrain can result in frontal headaches or even migraine-type headaches, especially when the work is associated with high expectations or perfectionism.

Overindulgence in sexual activities is another cause of headaches, especially for men. Dizziness after intercourse is a warning signal that perhaps sexual frequency should be tapered. Women who have had numerous childbirths can develop generalized or eye-related headaches.

Excessive physical activity, such as exercising or playing a sport, is another cause of headaches. In women, headaches related to this cause often manifest themselves during or after menstruation.

Western Treatment

Medication such as Tylenol for relief of symptoms during the headache; also (e.g., with migraine headaches) medication to help prevent the onset of an episode.

Chinese Treatment

For chronic, recurrent headaches, avoid the relevant problems in diet, emotions, or lifestyle that are described above. For any attack of an acute or chronic, recurrent headache, do the following, based on the particular location or nature of the headache:

- For a frontal headache (Yangming meridians): Massage LI 4, Yintang, ST 40, ST 44, and ST 45.
- For a temple or side headache (Shaoyang meridian): Massage in order TB 5, GB 41, Taiyang, and GB 20. Also massage LR 3, SP 6, KI 3, and LI 4. In addition, massage the N micromeridian on the inside of the palmar surface of the little finger; massage from the tip toward the palm.
- For a frontal headache: Massage DU 20, BL 10, BL 60, and

GB 20; if the headache is acute, also massage LU 7.

- For a parietal (top of head) headache (Jueyin meridian): Massage DU 20, LR 3, and BL 67.
- For a migraine headache (throbbing in temples, eyes, or sides of head, possibly accompanied by dizziness, irritability, bitter taste, red face, or visual effects, and often occurring in women before or during menstruation): Massage in sequence: TB 5, GB 41, and GB 20. Also can massage LR 2, LR 3, LI 4, LI 11, KI 3, and SP 6.
- For a generalized headache, associated with a feeling of heaviness: Massage LI 4, SP 3, CV 12, LU 7, and ST 40.
- For a nonmigraine headache accompanying menstruation (organized by time period):

  Before the period—a sharp headache in the temple, eyes, or side of head, usually in women whose periods have a lot of clots or are painful: Massage in sequence SP 4 and P 6, and then add the following points (sequential order not necessary): SP 6, LR 3, DU 20, and SP 10.

  Before or during the period—a migraine headache: see above, "For a migraine headache."

  During or after the period—a dull, achy headache at the top of the head with, possibly, dizziness, insomnia, fatigue, paleness, or heart palpitations: Massage in sequence LU 7 and KI 6, then add the following points (sequential order not necessary): CV 4, ST 36, SP 6, and BL 20.

Hemorrhoids

Symptoms

Itchiness and discomfort of the anus, becoming painful when sitting; sometimes accompanied by protrusion ("prolapse") of blood vessels from the anus, bleeding (usually bright red), and/or constipation (with hard stools).

Description

Essentially, hemorrhoids are clumps of normal blood vessels present in everyone. There are two types: internal (located deep within the rectum) and external (located at, or close to, the anus). Problems occur when these vessels become enlarged.

Common causes of hemorrhoids include chronic constipation; increased pressure on the liver (portal) blood vessels; and, in pregnant women, increased pressure on the rectal and anal blood vessels.

In Chinese medicine, hemorrhoids are the result of a Spleen Qi deficiency. The proper direction for Spleen Qi is upward, creating a "lifting" effect along the midline of the body that holds organs and structures in place. When Spleen Qi is disturbed, there may be a prolapse of organs or structures, such as rectal or anal hemorrhoids.

Spleen Qi also keeps blood in the blood vessels, so deficient Spleen Qi can cause the bleeding associated with hemorrhoids. Furthermore, Spleen Qi is Digestive Qi, so Spleen Qi abnormality can lead to the kind of chronic constipation that produces hemorrhoids.

Western Treatment

At home, external hemorrhoids can be treated with over-the-counter shrinking medications. Also, constipation-related symptoms and causes of hemorrhoids in general can be alleviated with a high-fiber diet and stool softeners.

In some cases, professional treatment may be necessary. Among the options are: rubber band litigation (tying off hemorrhoids with rubber bands and therefore "starving" hemorrhoids of blood); electrical, laser, or infrared stimulation to coagulate blood and stop bleeding; or, infrequently, surgical incision to remove hemorrhoids.

Chinese Treatment

To tonify the Spleen, pull Qi upward, and address other hemorrhoid-related problems, do the following things as appropriate to the specific situation:

For general treatment of all hemorrhoid cases:
- Massage BL 57 and SP 3.
- Massage BL 20 or, alternatively, the midback in a clockwise motion.
- Massage DU 4 or, alternatively, the lower back in a clockwise motion.
- On the hand, massage the F micromeridian on the middle of the little finger, from the tip to the palm.
- Avoid cold and phlegm-producing foods and excessive intake of sugar/sweet foods.
- Keep the abdomen covered and warm; also rub the palms (the micro system correspondence for the abdomen) together to keep them warm.

If constipated, also massage SP 15.

If constipated and suffering from external hemorrhoids, add more massage of the lower back in a clockwise motion, to ensure more massage of the Large Intestine back Shu points.

In any case of external hemorrhoids, add the following:
- Massage the lower back more frequently, in a clockwise motion.
- Massage the groin close to the pubic area.
- Massage the crown of the head to stimulate DU 20 and to raise Qi upward.
- Massage CV 6.

If bleeding, massage SP 1.

Hiccups

Symptoms

An involuntary short, sharp breath or series of breaths producing a "hic"- or "hiccup"-like sound.

Description

Hiccups are produced by a spasm and sudden contraction of the diaphragm. During normal breathing, the diaphragm lowers on the "in" breath to move more air into the lungs, and rises on the "out" breath to expel air out of the lungs. When the diaphragm spasms, the movement of air into the lungs is rushed. This causes the glottis, or "door" of the airway, to close abruptly and the vocal cords to vibrate rapidly with a "hic"/"hiccup" sound.

Usually hiccups occur randomly in a short-lasting series that is physiologically normal. A rare case of hiccups may continue for days, weeks, or even longer. The cause of such a serious case may be a hereditary tendency toward hiccuping aggravated by an irritation of the diaphragm due to a lung disease, a gastrointestinal disorder, alcoholism, a metabolic problem, or a tumor.

In Chinese medicine, a hiccup is another possible result of rebellious Stomach Qi: it moves upward instead of downward (the proper direction), making it impossible for Lung Qi to descend. The cause of the Stomach Qi disruption can be any Lung or gastrointestinal problem or any illness that indirectly affects the Lung or the Stomach.

Western Treatment

Left alone, the hiccups usually will disappear in minutes. Possible home remedies include holding one's breath as long as possible; experiencing a sudden fright; breathing in and out of a paper bag (a confined space); eating dry, granulated sugar; drinking a cold liquid; and so on.

Rare cases of longer-lasting hiccups may require professional treatment to avoid or alleviate exhaustion. The treatment may take the form of drugs, stimulation of the phrenic nerve (which innervates the diaphragm), or, infrequently, surgery to crush the phrenic nerve. Professional testing also is advisable in such cases to identify any underlying illnesses that may need treatment.

Chinese Treatment

For relief from a sudden attack of hiccups, massage P 6, LU 9, and ST 36. For more persistent cases, consult a physician.

Hives

Symptoms

Skin lesions that form a specific pattern known as "wheal and flare," characterized by a raised, irregular border; may be red or pale, itchy, and/or warm to the touch.

Description

In Western medicine, hives are associated with allergic reaction. They can be localized in the area of contact with the allergy-causing substance, or they can be generalized when the person is exposed to an airborne or food-triggered allergen.

In Chinese medicine, localized hives are caused by an internal Damp Heat condition that makes the skin more vulnerable when it comes in contact with an allergy-causing substance. Generalized hives can be associated with a Wind invasion; the specific problem involved may be either an external pathogen or a harmful emotion, especially frustration, anger, or irritability. See *Eczema* in this guide for more information about hives and related skin conditions.

Western Treatment

When the hives are in a small, localized area, they many need only topical steroid cream application. More systemic, generalized, or multisited hives need oral antihistamines; and sometimes, in severe cases, short-term oral steroids.

Chinese Treatment

Chinese treatment varies according to whether the condition is Wind Cold, characterized by pale lesions that get worse when exposed to the wind or cold, or Wind Heat, characterized by lesions that are red, hot, and itchy. Recurrent hives are associated with persistent internal dampness and heat and may be brought on by adverse emotions.

For Wind Cold hives, massage GB 20, ST 36, LU 5, and SP 10. Also, avoid cold foods.

For Wind Heat hives, massage the same points as for Wind Cold (see above), and add LI 11 and LR 8.

For recurrent hives, add ST 40 and SP 6. Also avoid situations that invoke frustration, irritability, or anger, or teach yourself new ways to respond to such situations that don't give rise to the same harmful emotions.

Hypertension (High Blood Pressure)

Symptoms (when present; usually no symptoms)

Headache, dizziness, eyesight changes; in children and infants, irritability and waking up frequently at night. (For other symptoms, see below under "Chinese Treatment.")

Description

In Western medicine, hypertension, or high blood pressure (HBP), is a condition of significantly greater than normal pressure on the arterial walls caused by the pumping action of the heart, the volume of blood, and the sympathetic nervous system controlling the diameter of the blood vessels. It is known as a silent killer because the majority of people who have it don't feel or observe any symptoms until it causes life-threatening heart disease or a stroke.

Typically hypertension is detected in the course of a routine checkup, where it manifests as a resting pressure of 160/95 or higher. Among adults, the standard measurement is 120/80 at age thirty and 140/85 at age forty and over (women tend to have lower blood pressure than men) Among children, normal blood pressure varies with age, height, weight, gender, and stage of puberty. Since blood pressure fluctuates with body position, time of day, physical activity, and mental state, a diagnosis should not be made with just one reading.

In most cases the actual cause of hypertension is not identifiable, so it is called essential hypertension or primary hypertension. Other cases, labeled secondary hypertension, can be attributed to a specific cause such as renal disease (renal hypertension); adrenal disease (adrenal hypertension); hormonal imbalances (e.g., from hormone-secreting tumors or oral contraceptives;) anatomical abnormalities; exposure to toxins (e.g., from cigarette smoking); or emotional stress, especially when it involves anxiety or anger.

Like Western medicine, Chinese medicine attributes hypertension to problems in the complex network that controls blood flow. In Chinese terms, this network involves many different systems: the Heart, Kidneys, Master of the Heart meridian (analogous to the sympathetic nervous system), and the Liver—the main director of Qi and blood flow that's associated with the emotions of anxiety and anger.

Western Treatment

It is important for people with hypertension to consult a doctor so that possible causes can be identified or ruled out. Doctors prescribe specific programs of treatment to fit individual cases and, if applicable, their underlying causes. Hypertension itself can be treated with various medications. The most common are diuretics that increase salt and water excretion to lessen the load for the heart. Other medications act on the sympathetic nervous system's control of blood vessels or on the vessels themselves. At home, a low-salt diet and a low-stress schedule are advised.

Chinese Treatment

The treatment suggestions below should complement Western treatment rather than replace it. The blood pressure needs to be monitored regularly, and any adjustment of medication should be made only in consultation with a physician or an M.D./acupuncturist.

Treat the hypertension according to the best-fitting description of symptoms:

For hyperactivity of Liver Yang and Liver Qi (dizziness, insomnia, dreaminess, headache, fidgetiness, bitter taste in the mouth, worsening of symptoms with physical or emotional exertion, sometimes a painful sensation around the eyes):

- Massage LR 3, GB 20, TB 5, GB 41, and LI 11.
- Massage eye points BL 1 and GB 1.
- Avoid excess physical activity and emotional stress (especially anger or frustration).
- Do calming exercises (see chapter 5).
- Avoid excessive intake of drugs that may be toxic to the Liver—for example, Tylenol (read warnings on labels).

For a deficiency of Liver Yin and Kidney Yin (headache, dizziness, ear-ringing, feverish sensation in palms and soles of feet):

- Tonify the Liver by massaging LR 3 and LR 8.
- Tonify the Kidney by massaging BL 23 (or, alternatively, by rubbing the lower back in a clockwise motion) and KI 3.
- Avoid excess intake of salt and sour foods.

For a deficiency of Kidney Yang (edema [swelling], feeling cold, fatigue, depression, pale urine):

- Massage BL 23 (or, alternatively, the lower back in a clockwise motion).
- Tonify the Kidney by massaging KI 7.
- Massage ST 36 and LI 11.
- Massage CV 4 (or, alternatively, the lower abdomen— below the navel—in a clockwise motion).
- Avoid excess intake of salt, and get plenty of rest.

For a disturbance of Heart Qi (palpitations, insomnia, dizziness, headaches, ear-ringing):

- Calm and regulate the Heart by massaging HT 7 and P 6.
- Massage Anmian, Yintang, LI 4, and LI 11.
- Avoid excessive intake of bitter-tasting foods—for example, bitter chocolate.
- Do calming exercises (see chapter 5).

For stagnation of phlegm in the Head (heavy sensation in the Head, dizziness, nausea, full feeling in the chest and abdomen):
- Massage ST 40, ST 36, LI 4, LI 11, and SP 6.
- Avoid excessive intake of phlegm-producing foods and sweets.

Impetigo

Symptoms

Red areas of skin that have a weepy, sometimes puslike discharge. *Note:* When the redness has a streak that leads away from the infected area, this means that the infection is spreading into a condition called cellulitis and should immediately be seen by a doctor.

Description

In Western medical terms, impetigo usually is an acute infection of the skin secondary to diaper rash, eczema, or any cut or scrape. In Chinese medical terms, it is associated with a Damp Heat condition that may be an acute situation or a buildup from previous illnesses, from weak Spleen Qi, or from a faulty diet. A sallow or slightly yellowish facial complexion is often associated with internal Damp Heat.

Western Treatment

Antibiotic ointment; in severe cases, oral antibiotics.

Chinese Treatment

Massage LU 5, LI 11, ST 40, and SP 10. Also, avoid foods that produce excess phlegm or heat.

Insomnia (Sleep Problems)

Symptoms

Insufficient sleep at night due to an inability to fall asleep; or a tendency to fall asleep easily but then to wake up several times during the night; early waking and being unable to fall back asleep. Any of these conditions may be accompanied by upsetting dreams; nightmares; or, in the case of children, attacks of "night terror" (sudden, panicky, apparently nondream-related awakening, often attributable to emotional trauma or a developmental conflict).

Description

According to Western medicine, the sleeping body goes into a general state of lesser activity (hypometabolism) that includes a lowering of the heart and breathing rates, of the secretion of hormones, of body temperature, and so on. There are several different stages of sleep characterized by different signs. For example, dreaming occurs during the rapid-eye-movement (REM) stage of sleep, which also has other changes, such as irregular heart and breathing rates, low muscle tone, and so on. Men sometimes experience penile erection during REM sleep.

Sleep is considered necessary to help the body restore its metabolic and brain functions. The required amount of sleep varies from person to person, but it is generally accepted that everyone needs several hours each night to function well the next day.

There are many different causes of insomnia. The physical ones include pain of any kind; internal diseases, such as diabetes; hormone imbalances, such as hyperthyroidism; excess consumption of caffeinated drinks; excess activity before bedtime; irregular sleep patterns, such as napping during the day; and jet lag. Insomnia also can be caused by emotional or psychological factors, the most common being anxiety, depression, and stress.

Chinese medicine distinguishes among numerous types of insomnia, described below under "Chinese Treatment," and which relate in different ways to dreams, diet, work habits, and emotions that can lead to excess or deficiency states. Some of these imbalances directly or indirectly affect the Heart, so the Heart is frequently included in Chinese treatment guidelines.

Sleep at night is the necessary Yin cycle of inactivity to balance the Yang cycle of activity during the day. Yang cannot function well when Yin is out of balance, and vice versa. This is comparable to the Western notion that sleep helps to restore metabolic and brain functions.

Western Treatment

In consultation with a doctor, the insomniac needs to evaluate and identify underlying causes of the condition and treat them accordingly. For example, it may be advisable to eliminate decaffeinated drinks in the evening, take medications for pain, or gain better control over diabetes or hyperthyroidism.

It's generally a good idea not to drink alcohol late in the evening, as some people fall asleep after drinking but wake up in two or three hours. Other commonsense, prebedtime approaches include relaxing (e.g., by avoiding violent TV shows), taking a warm bath, or drinking a warm glass of milk.

Medications include both over-the-counter or prescription tranquilizers and sleeping pills such as barbiturates. Antidepressants and psychotherapy are often prescribed when insomnia is thought to be emotional or psychological in origin.

Chinese Treatment

For any kind of insomnia, massage Yintang, Anmian, HT 7, KI 6, and BL 1. Also, read through the following descriptions/

225

treatments for excess and deficiency states, choose the one that best fits the situation, and apply the corresponding treatment.

The following descriptions/treatments are for excess states, characterized in general by restless sleep and sometimes by an inability to sleep on one's back:

Waking up during the night with mental and/or physical restlessness, sometimes accompanied by a stuffy sensation in the chest, dreams with flying images, heart palpitations, excess worrying:

- Massage HT 7 and HT 8 together.
- Massage Anmian, Yintang, and CV 15.
- Meditate or engage in other peaceful activities to calm the mind. It's most important to do this before bedtime, but it also needs to be done throughout the day so the mind is not all wound up and difficult to unwind when retiring.
- Avoid excessive intake of bitter foods.

Restless sleep with a lot of tossing and turning, unpleasant dreams, heavy-feeling body during the day, poor appetite:

- Massage Anmian, HT 7, ST 36, ST 40, SP 6, and the midback in a clockwise direction to tonify the digestive Spleen Qi.
- Massage the F micromeridian on the hand: the middle of the fifth finger, palm side, from the tip to the palm.
- Avoid phlegm-producing foods and excessive intake of sweets.

Restlessness with irritability, headaches, anger, depression, nightmares:

- Massage Anmian, LR 3, GB 44, HT 7, and Yintang.
- Massage the midback clockwise.
- Be more aware of situations that cause irritability, headaches, anger, or depression, and control these responses through meditation or other calming activities.
- Avoid excessive intake of sour foods.

The following descriptions/treatments are for deficiency states, characterized in general by problematic sleep rhythms:

Difficulty falling asleep, excessive worry, heart palpitations, fatigue, poor appetite, poor memory, pale complexion:
- Massage HT 7, SP 6, ST 36, and Anmian.
- Massage the upper back and midback in a clockwise direction to tonify the Heart and the digestive system.

Waking up frequently, restlessness, night sweats, forgetfulness, feeling of heat:
- Massage HT 7, KI 3, KI 6, SP 6, ST 36, and Anmian.
- Massage the lower back in a clockwise direction.
- Avoid excessive work and take more time for relaxation.

Waking up early and not being able to fall back asleep, fearfulness, light sleep, many dreams, easily startled, lack of motivation and initiative, inability to be assertive, fatigue:
- Massage Anmian, Yintang, HT 7, GB 40, and KI 3.
- Massage the lower back in a clockwise direction.

Waking during the night, many dreams, sleeptalking, sleepwalking, irritability, dry eyes or other eye complains, dilated pupils. (*Note:* These are frequent symptoms among children with insomnia, who may also go through night terror, appear frightened and/or confused, and experience faster breathing and heart rates.):
- Massage Anmian, Yintang, HT 7, LR 3, SP 6, and BL 1.
- Massage the upper back and midback clockwise in a large circle to include the outer half of the back.
- Massage the F micromeridian on the fifth finger, middle channel, from the tip toward the palm.

Jaundice, Newborn

Note: Jaundice or suspected jaundice in older children and adults (most commonly associated with hepatitis and sometimes, in adults, with cancer or cirrhosis) is a complicated condition that varies greatly from person to person. It requires immediate attention by a physician. Acupuncture has often proved to be a helpful treatment.

Symptoms

Yellowish eyes and skin and yellower urine, usually during the first week of life but, in some breast-fed babies, continuing for as long as three weeks.

Description

Newborn jaundice, indicating an excess accumulation of bilirubin in the bloodstream, occurs in approximately 75 percent of newborns. In most cases it is a temporary, benign condition that Western medicine calls "physiologic jaundice." As the baby adjusts from the fetal stage (when bilirubin is eliminated by the mother's placenta) to the independent stage (when bilirubin is eliminated by the baby's liver), the escalating breakdown of red blood cells causes an increase in bilirubin production.

Physiologic jaundice usually occurs within the first two to three days of a full-term newborn (sooner in premature infants) and disappears by one week of age. A small percentage of breast-fed babies may develop jaundice from a hormone in the milk that interferes with bilirubin metabolism. This jaundice usually occurs during the second half of the first week of life and continues for two to three weeks.

Other, less common causes of prolonged jaundice include infection, incompatibility and disorders, congenital malformations, and neonatal hepatitis. All pediatricians routinely perform laboratory studies in newborns with jaundice so that the more serious conditions are ruled out.

The Chinese explanation for the major cause of newborn jaundice corresponds very closely to the Western one. From a Chinese perspective, physiologic jaundice is a sign that the baby has a Yang deficiency due to an immature Yang physiology—the Liver and Gallbladder being unable to maintain a free flow of Qi.

Western Treatment

For physiologic jaundice, give the baby extra water to help bilirubin excretion, and place him or her in sunlight (or under "bililights"), since lights help convert bilirubin into a substance more easily excreted by the kidney. For newborn jaundice due to breast-feeding, continue breast-feeding, but increase the baby's water intake, and place him or her in sunlight.

Chinese Treatment

Massage the following areas and points to strengthen the baby's Liver-Gallbladder system and to increase excretion:
- using the palms: the inside of each lower leg, upward from the ankle to the knee; and the outside of each lower leg, downward from the knee to the ankle
- the middle and lower back separately, in small, clockwise circles
- LR 3, KI 3, SP 6, and LI 11

Also, give the baby extra water and place him or her in sunlight.

Jet Lag

Symptoms

Light-headedness, irritability, confusion, change in appetite, digestive disturbances, fatigue, insomnia.

Description

Jet lag can occur when traveling by air across time zones so that the destination's time zone is significantly different from the time zone of departure. Such travel can disrupt one's biological and physiological rhythms—in common language, one's "body clock." The more time zones the traveler crosses, the more severe the symptoms and the more time needed for readjustment. Jet lag tends to be less troublesome when traveling from east to west: time is "gained" by going in this direction, and it is easier for the body to adapt to a longer day than to a shorter one.

Like Western medicine, Chinese medicine recognizes the adverse impact on the body and mind caused by sudden physical relocation in another time zone. In Chinese medicine, the human body is a microcosm of the natural world, and it is highly important to follow the rhythms of the natural world to maintain good health. When these rhythms are abruptly altered in an "unnatural" way (jet flight), one's health may simultaneously be affected.

Qi flow in the body as a whole follows the rhythm of day and night: maximum Yang Qi during the day and maximum Yin Qi during the night. Meanwhile, Qi flow in individual organs follows two-hour rhythms: for example, Lung Qi is strongest between 3 A.M. and 5 A.M. and weakest between 3 P.M. and 5 P.M., while Stomach Qi is strongest between 7 A.M. and 9 A.M. and weakest between 7 P.M. and 9 P.M. When one's eating and sleeping schedule is radically altered—by either jet lag or a work-shift change—the body winds up performing its normal functions at inappropriate times: for example, digesting breakfast in what, under normal circumstances, is the middle of the night, or, in other words, performing a Yang activity during a Yin cycle.

Western Treatment

If possible, gradually ease from one schedule into another with a period of minor adjustment before and after traveling. For example, suppose that the travel is from California to New York—a three-hour jump ahead in time. A day or two *before* leaving, eat meals one hour earlier than usual (say, 5 P.M. PST instead of 6 P.M. PST). A day or two *after* arriving, eat meals one hour later than usual (say, 7 P.M. EST instead of 6 P.M. EST). Follow the same process with bedtime.

A possible treatment for insomnia due to jet lag is taking a melatonin supplement. Melatonin is a hormone secreted by the pineal gland that is thought to help induce sleep.

Chinese Treatment

In addition to the gradual conditioning process described above (see "Western Treatment"), do the following things to make a smoother general adjustment from one time zone to another:

- Massage the Yintang point.
- Avoid stimulatory food and drink (e.g., caffeinated beverages), and drugs or alcohol that induce drowsiness.

To treat insomnia as a result of jet lag, do the following:

- Massage the midforehead at the hairline and the bottom of the flap of skin in front of the ear. Both of these points correspond to the pineal gland.
- Massage KI 6 to stimulate Yin Qi, then BL 1 to "close" the eyes.

To induce wakefulness while jet-lagged, massage BL 62 to stimulate Yang Qi, followed by BL 1 to "open" the eyes.

To increase Digestive Qi while jet-lagged, massage SP 6, ST 36, and the F micromeridian channel on the hand—the middle of the fifth finger, massage from the tip toward the palm.

Menstrual Problems

Symptoms

Any of the following: unusually heavy or light bleeding; menstrual pain, usually in the lower abdominal area; increased or decreased frequency or nonoccurrence of periods; emotional distress; headache.

Description

Western medicine attributes most menstrual problems to hormonal imbalance, physical abnormalities, or emotional stress. Normal menstruation is defined as lasting from three to seven days and occurring every twenty-one to thirty-six days. Normal flow is characterized as light in volume and pale red at the beginning of the period; heavy and dark red during the middle; and light and pink toward the end.

From a Chinese standpoint, normal menstruation lasts four to six days and occurs every twenty-six to thirty-two days; but more emphasis is placed on the *regularity* of periods. Several different organs or body systems have a special connection with menstruation, and women are very vulnerable to health risks or imbalances during menstruation. Here are the various contributing factors that could be involved (treatment varies according to factor):

Climate or external influences
- Cold: During menstruation (and after childbirth), cold can easily enter the uterus and result in a painful period (dysmenorrhea).
- Damp: Dampness can come up from the feet and legs into the ovaries and uterus, causing a painful period. When dampness combines with heat, symptoms of infection can occur, such as vaginal discharges.
- Heat: Excess heat can cause heavy menstrual bleeding.

Emotional stress
- Sadness or depression can affect the Heart, which governs the circulation of blood. In such cases, the period flow man be scanty, delayed, or even missed (amenorrhea).
- Worry tends to knot up Qi, which can lead to Qi stagnation, resulting in delayed or painful periods. Sometimes additional signs include a tight feeling in the chest, breast distension, and/or premenstrual-syndrome (PMS) symptoms, such as increased irritability or mood swings.

  A more serious, chronic state of fear or anxiety can result in a Qi deficiency that causes many different kinds of gynecological disorders. Shock can trigger a delay of the menstrual cycle and even a missed period.
- Anger or frustration can stagnate Qi and cause irregular

periods, clotting, PMS symptoms, painful menstruation, lower abdominal pain, and/or a bloated feeling.

- Long-standing guilt or self-blame can cause a sinking of Qi, which can lead to a feeling of heaviness or dysfunction in the organs of the lower abdomen, such as the Bladder and/or uterus. The result may be menstrual problems. Bladder symptoms may include urinary incontinence or frequent urination.

Diet

- Excessive intake of cold foods may produce a problematic coldness in the uterus (e.g., a small amount of salad may be nutritious, but a large amount may not be). The most vulnerable periods for this kind of effect are during puberty, during menstruation, and right after childbirth.
- Excessive intake of hot foods can cause painful periods.
- Very restrictive diets (e.g., vegetarian or high-protein) can lead to scanty periods, missed periods, or even infertility.
- Excessive intake of greasy foods can cause vaginal discharge and/or painful periods.

Physical/mental activity

- Excessive work or exercise can cause Qi and blood stagnation, leading to painful periods. Girls during puberty are especially vulnerable, given their tendency to engage in sports activities, to go out more often into the cold (another cause of Qi stagnation), and to wear scanty clothing (such as shorts), thereby exposing more of their body to the cold. Excessive work or exercise during menstruation increases the risk of having a painful period.
- Excessive sexual activity can deplete a woman's Qi and lead to missed periods, scanty periods, or a delay in the menstrual cycle. A woman is especially vulnerable to these effects during the early teen years. The timing of sex is also important. Sex during a menstrual period can result in

a clashing of blood flowing downward vs. sperm moving upward, thus causing physical pain. Sex shortly after menstruation, which reopens the cervix, may induce further bleeding.

Chinese medical treatment also varies according to different major kinds of menstrual problems:

Frequent menstruation (polymenorrhea)—more periods per year, with a shorter cycle for each period:
- Heat type: indicated by a heavy, red menstrual flow and a restless, dry feeling.
- Qi deficiency type: characterized by a lighter-colored flow early in the period, palpitations, dizziness, poor appetite, and soft stools.
- Cold type: indicated by a delayed cycle, blood clots, a menstrual flow that is not smooth, and lower abdominal pain following intake of cold foods.
- Blood-deficient type: features a delayed cycle; a scanty, thin menstrual flow; palpitations; tiredness; and dizziness.

Painful menstruation (dysmenorrhea)
- Excessive type: indicated by scanty, purple menstrual flow; depression; feeling of bloatedness in the sides.
- Deficient type: indicated either by a scanty flow with abdominal pain; or by slight abdominal pain before the flow, vaginal discharge, and dizziness.

Nonoccurrence of period (amenorrhea): characterized by many different deficiency conditions and stagnation syndromes.

Western Treatment

Directed toward specific hormone therapy (e.g., to correct a thyroid imbalance) and/or treatment of physical abnormalities (e.g., ovarian cysts). In some cases when no other symptom can be identified, emotional stress is diagnosed and treated.

Chinese Treatment

For frequent menstruation:
- Heat type: Massage LR 3, KI 3, CV 4, SP 6, and LI 11. Also avoid hot, greasy, and spicy foods.
- Deficiency type: Massage ST 36, KI 3, CV 4, and SP 6. Also avoid overworking.
- Cold type: Massage DU 4 Mingmen, ST 29, CV 4, KI 3, and ST 36. Also avoid cold foods and dairy products, and keep the lower abdomen warm.
- Blood-deficient type: Massage ST 36, BL 20, CV 4, and SP 6.

For painful menstruation:
- Excessive type: Massage CV 3, CV 4, SP 6, CV 12, and the lower abdomen clockwise. Also avoid cold foods.
- Deficient type: For a scanty period with abdominal pain, massage CV 4, SP 6, BL 18, BL 20, and the midback clockwise. For slight abdominal pain before the onset of the period, vaginal discharge, or dizziness, massage CV 4, SP 6, KI 3, BL 23, and the lower back clockwise.

For nonoccurrence of period, consult a health professional and also do the following:
- Massage the midback and the lower back clockwise to tonify the body. These two parts of the back can be massaged sequentially or simultaneously (by using both hands), depending on the skill or the comfort of the person doing the massage.
- Massage the lower abdomen clockwise
- Massage KI 3, KI 6, LU 7, ST 36, SP 6, LR 8, and LR 3.
- Massage the J micromeridian on the back side of the fifth finger, along the lateral/outer border, from the tip to the palm.
- Massage the N micromeridian, palm-side surface of the fifth finger, along the side next to the fourth finger; and

the F micromeridian, in the middle of the fifth finger—
massage both from the tip to the palm.

Also do the following, as appropriate:
* For all menstrual problems: Review the "Diet" and "Phys-
ical/mental activity" sections above. Avoid the excesses
and imbalances indicated.
* For alleviating anger or frustration: Massage CV 4, LR 3,
and P 6.
* For counteracting the effects of excessive sexual activity:
Massage DU 4 Mingmen, BL 23, KI 3, CV 4, ST 36, and
SP 6.
* For alleviating headache associated with menstruation, see
appropriate guidelines under *Headache* in this guide.

Motion Sickness

Symptoms
Dizziness, nausea.

Description
In Western medicine, motion sickness is explained in
anatomical terms as an overload of signals to the structures in
the inner ear that give a person a sense of balance. While some
people (e.g., fans of roller coasters) enjoy the surprise of sudden
changes in horizontal or vertical orientation, others suffer
adverse physical reactions. Common triggers of motion sickness
are rides in boats (seasickness), planes (airsickness), and cars (car-
sickness), all of which subject the passenger to vertical dipping
and horizontal swaying.

Chinese medicine theorizes that sudden changes in vertical
and/or horizontal direction result in a disturbance of Qi flow
that creates "rebellious Qi"—Qi that flows in the opposite direction from normal.

Western Treatment

Motion sickness is commonly treated with medications such as Dramamine (an antihistamine) and Transderm scop (a skin patch that releases scopalamine into the bloodstream). The precise action of Dramamine is not known, but the skin patch probably works on the central nervous system's response to sensory stimuli from motion. Both medications can cause drowsiness.

Chinese Treatment

To regulate the Qi flow and help prevent or alleviate motion sickness, do the following:

* Massage P6, the biggest point for nausea from any cause, including morning sickness during pregnancy.
* Massage ST 36 and LR 3.
* Massage CV 12: either the point or the whole CV 12 area clockwise.
* Massage the E micromeridian for the Stomach: on the lateral border of the palm side of the fifth finger, from the tip toward the palm.

Nervous Stomach

(also see *Abdominal Pain* and *Gastritis*)

Symptoms

A sensation of having knots in the stomach that's associated with being nervous (i.e., restless, uneasy, irritable, and/or hyperexcitable); may be accompanied by disturbances in sleeping, eating, or drinking habits and feelings of being overwhelmed or threatened by personal problems.

Description

In Western medicine, nervous stomach is generally due to emotional stress and/or a poor diet or dietary habits.

In Chinese medicine, nervous Stomach is one of a number of illnesses causing or resulting from excess heat in the Stomach. It may be related to a diet of too many hot, fried, or phlegm-pro-ducing foods or to emotional upset.

Western Treatment

In consultation with a doctor, identify the stressful life situa-tions or factors that may be causing nervous stomach and the steps that can be taken to alleviate them. Professional counseling and/or medications to decrease nervousness may be prescribed.

Chinese Treatment

Massage the following:
* the middle burner above the navel clockwise
* ST 44, ST 45, SP 6, CV 12, and P 6

Also, do calming exercises and mediation (see chapter 5), and avoid stressful situations.

Nosebleed (Epistaxis)

Symptoms

Bleeding from the nostrils.

Description

Nosebleeds are most common in young children, with a decreased rate of incidence after puberty. Isolated episodes usu-ally can be attributed to trauma (such as a blow to the nose), nose-picking, foreign bodies in the nose, respiratory infections, or allergies. Recurrent nosebleeds point to an anatomical prob-lem (e.g., a nasal polyp), a bleeding disorder, or some other chronic problem (such as high blood pressure).

Chinese medicine recognizes these causes and also posits another one: the absorption of an external heat pathogen that results in a drying out of the nasal membranes. This explanation correlates to the Western concept of a respiratory infection. Recurrent nosebleeds usually are attributed to internal Heat accu-mulation, most commonly in the Lung channel (the nose is the external orifice for this channel) or the Stomach channel (which has a branch going to the sinuses).

Western Treatment

Apply pressure to the nose to stop the bleeding. Serious cases may require professional cauterization followed by application of a nasal pack. In persistent or serious cases, consult a physician to rule out, among other things, a bleeding disorder that may need transfusions.

If the nosebleed is associated with an acute infection, the infection itself needs to be treated. To help prevent nosebleeds related to chronic conditions such as a nasal polyp or a bleeding disorder or to chronic illnesses such as high blood pressure, run a humidifier in commonly used rooms to prevent environmental dryness, which can help to trigger nosebleeds.

Chinese Treatment

In addition to applying pressure or a nasal pack to the nose, do the following:
- For acute bleeding, pinch hard on SP 1.
- Massage LI 20 to alleviate acute bleeding and to prevent future nosebleeds.
- Massage LI 11, LU 5, LI 4, and ST 44 to clear Heat from the system.
- Avoid "hot" foods.

Obesity

Symptoms

Excessive body fat, sometimes accompanied by physical illnesses related to being overly heavy, including gallstones, high blood pressure, strokes, diabetes, cardiovascular problems, respiratory problems (such as difficulty breathing), hormone imbalances, and even some forms of cancer.

239

Description

Fat is a good source of energy and provides protection for internal organs. Too much fat, however, predisposes a person not only to certain physical illnesses (mentioned above under "Symptoms") but also to various interpersonal and psychological problems. In a culture where slimness is a standard of beauty, fat people are often ridiculed for their appearance, unfairly stereo-typed (e.g., as gluttons), or discriminated against in jobs and social situations. The result is an erosion of self-esteem and self-confidence.

It can be difficult to draw a clear line between being over-weight and being obese (or *excessively* overweight). Physicians often define obesity as having a body mass index (BMI) of 27 or above, referring to a person's weight in kilograms divided by his or her height in meters: the larger the quotient beyond 27, the more excessive the weight. In fact, many people whose BMI falls below 27 still can be considered obese if their weight poses strong physical or emotional risks or problems.

Although overeating does contribute to the development of obesity, recent studies show that the cause of obesity for many people is not too much food but too little fat-burning activity. Obesity also can be associated with heredity; with hormone imbalances (e.g., due to hypothyroidism); with disorders of the hypothalamus gland, which regulates appetite; and with emo-tional problems that, for various reasons, prompt one to seek solace, self-gratification, or self-fortification in food. Another contributing factor may be the use of drugs, such as steroids or antidepressant medications.

Chinese medicine offers several explanations of obesity that are comparable to Western ones. Both agree that obesity involves a disturbance in the digestive system. In Chinese terms, food goes to the Stomach, where "ripening and rotting" normally occur (comparable to what Westerners understand as the break-down of food by enzymes). The Spleen/Pancreas system then does its normal job of transforming food into Nutritive Qi that the body uses as energy. When Stomach Qi is deficient, food breakdown is impaired. When Spleen Qi is deficient, the transformation of food into Nutritive Qi is compromised. As a result of either or both problems, food stagnates and is not properly "used," which is comparable to the Western notion of calories/fat not being "burned."

The Stomach does not function well with dryness, nor the Spleen/Pancreas with dampness. In addition, both organs/energy channels can be adversely affected by coldness and sweetness. As a result, warm soup, for example, helps with digestion, while cold, dry foods impair it. Phlegm-producing, sweet, and greasy/hot (drying) foods also interfere with normal digestive functioning. So can drugs: antibiotics are considered cold to the system, and antidepressants are thought to scatter needed Yang energy. Another impairing factor is a history of recent illnesses with fever, which can dry up fluid in the body as a whole, including the Stomach.

Both Chinese and Western medicine also recognize the significant role in obesity that can be played by mental and emotional turmoil. In Chinese terms, excessive thinking and worrying can lead to a Digestive Qi deficiency. Anger, frustration, and other kinds of emotional distress can cause Qi to stagnate, which also can lead to Digestive Qi problems. In addition, people under stress tend to ignore good diet practices—eating too much, too little, too fast, too irregularly, or too distractedly.

Finally, Chinese experts, like their Western counterparts, recognize the influence that lifestyle and heredity can have on obesity. In Chinese terms, too much work can deplete Qi so that less is available for proper digestion, while too little physical activity can result in sluggish Qi movement in general. Obesity also can represent a problem in Kidney Essence, which is passed down through the generations.

Western Treatment

Because of the numerous, serious problems associated with obesity and the consequent need for a professional and systematic treatment program, it is important to consult a physician. Some causes of obesity, such as hypothyroidism, can be medically treated. In any case, the individual needs to be tested for possible contributing or developing illnesses.

The mainstay of all effective weight management programs is a balanced regimen of diet and exercise supplemented by behavioral therapy (guidance in motivating oneself and acquiring healthier eating and lifestyle habits). For specific diet and exercise plans, follow a physician's advice relative to your particular situation.

Bear in mind that exercise alone rarely results in weight loss. Although it burns calories, it doesn't change the resting metabolic rate, which determines how quickly and effectively food is processed. On the other hand, diet alone does not work as quickly to reduce weight, and it does not provide the muscle-toning that keeps body tissues from progressively sagging as weight is lost.

Medication is another possible component of a weight loss program. Most prescribed drugs, such as amphetamines, act on the central nervous system to decrease appetite. Other drugs include those that act on the gastrointestinal tract, such as enzyme inhibitors, and various hormones. The drugs themselves do not increase weight loss but rather predispose the person to eat less. Unfortunately, there may be uncomfortable side effects, and weight gain is common after drug use is discontinued.

Surgical measures, advisable only in the most extreme cases of obesity, range from optional, cosmetic surgery (liposuction for fat removal) to various stomach reduction or intestinal bypass procedures. Possible complications of the more serious forms of surgery include liver disease, vitamin deficiencies, diarrhea, gallstones, and assorted intestinal problems.

Chinese Treatment

Like Western doctors, Chinese doctors recommend consulting a physician and following a program of proper diet, exercise, and lifestyle habits. As part of this program, the following things are advised:

Keep the abdomen, especially the navel, warm.

For food and eating:

- Avoid the following foods or liquids: anything that is chilled, frozen, or iced; raw fruits and vegetables, including salads; phlegm-producing foods, such as diary products, sugar, peanuts, or pork; alcohol (drying); sweet-greasy foods; and hot foods.

- Choose foods that are warm. Eat foods at room temperature or cooked.

- Put smaller portions of food on the plate, or divide the food on the plate into smaller portions (e.g, cut sandwiches into halves or fourths). People tend to eat an entire portion of food whether or not they're really hungry for it, so smaller or divided portions help prevent overeating.

- Schedule eating times when it's appropriate for optimum digestion. Stomach Qi is strongest from 7 A.M. to 9 A.M. and weakest from 7 P.M. to 9 P.M. Spleen Qi is strongest from 9 A.M. to 11 A.M. and weakest from 9 P.M. to 11 P.M. Therefore it's best to eat a hearty breakfast at about 7 A.M., a healthy lunch at about 11 A.M., a light dinner at about 6 P.M., and nothing after 9 P.M. Eating late at night is especially unhealthy because it stirs up Qi just when the body should be preparing for rest (the Yin cycle of less activity and sleep).

- Avoid eating too much (because Stomach Qi can't keep up with the demand) or too little (because it's not nutritious in general). Also avoid skipping meals.

- Avoid eating in a hurry, such as grabbing a hamburger on

the go or working immediately after eating. This does not allow the proper time for Digestive Qi to do its best work. Also avoid distractions while eating, such as working, watching TV, or reading. Intellectual activities diminish the Qi necessary for proper digestion.

- Avoid eating at irregular intervals or being inconsistent in the types of foods eaten (e.g., rich foods one day, salads the next). Each of these habits disrupts the regularity and rhythm of digestion.

Be sure to incorporate balanced amounts of work, place, and relaxation into the daily schedule (see chapter 5 for meditative relaxation suggestions).

For any accompanying emotional difficulties (such as depression or anxiety), see *Emotional Problems* in this guide and follow the appropriate guidelines.

Massage the following:
- SP 3, SP 4, and SP 6.
- CV 10 and CV 12.
- GB 8, the hypothalamus.
- the middle back in a circular, clockwise motion.

Pain
(includes ankle pain, arm pain, back pain, elbow pain, finger pain, hip pain, knee pain, shoulder pain, and wrist pain)

Note: For any of these pains, please read this entire entry up to "Chinese Treatment." Then, in "Chinese Treatment," read the general introduction followed by the section that offers guidelines for the particular kind of pain being experienced.

Symptoms

An unpleasant sensory and emotional experience, usually associated with actual or potential tissue damage; depending on the specific tissue or damage involved, the physical pain may be

244

dull or sharp; steady, throbbing, or intermittent; stinging, burning, or freezing; diffuse or localized.

Description

It's important to note that pain has both a physical and an
emotional component. Anger, anxiety, depression, fear, frustration, and other so-called negative emotions not only can generate pain on their own (medically defined as "psychosomatic"),
but also intensify pain that already exists.

Even pain itself, apart from what causes it, tends to be experienced emotionally as something bad, thus making the individual feel more sensitive to it and, ultimately, more physically
bothered by it. In some cases physical pain may lead to emotional illness, although such an outcome also may result from situational factors, such as living a more restricted, challenging, or
precarious life due to illness.

According to Western medicine, physical pain begins in the
form of signals from nerve receptors at the site. The signals
travel along one of two different kinds of nerve fibers to the
brain: one fiber, associated with dull, achy, nagging pain, transmits slowly; the other fiber, associated with acute, sharp pain,
transmits quickly. Other kinds of pain sensations are related to
the type of tissue involved and its location.

At times of pain, the body releases natural pain-control substances called endorphins (literally, "morphine within") that
often can reduce or eliminate the pain fairly soon, depending on
its cause and severity.

Chinese medicine defines pain as a complex symptom with a
variety of causes. In general, pain reflects an imbalance or disruption of the Qi flow in one or more channels, depending on
where in the body one feels the pain. This may explain why
some pains can't be scientifically (i.e., physically) traced; such
pains may occur only on an energetic (or Qi) level rather than on
a strictly physical level.

In Chinese terms, pain may result from either an excess condition or a deficient condition, as follows:

- *Excess condition:* Among the possible causes of an excess condition are the invasion of an external pathogen, such as wind or cold; an interior heat or coldness condition (such as a sore throat); the stagnation of Qi and blood; and the obstruction of Qi by phlegm, also resulting in food retention. All of these conditions are characterized by an obstruction of Qi flow in certain channels, which, in most cases, produces sharp pain. There is a familiar saying in Chinese medicine "If the channels are free, there is no pain. If the channels are blocked, there is pain."

- *Deficient condition:* Pain can be caused by a Qi and blood deficiency, as well as by a consumption of body fluids and consequent Yin deficiency. Certain channels become malnourished and, in most cases, produce a dull, achy pain.

Western Treatment

Anyone experiencing pain is strongly advised to consult a doctor to identify or rule out potential medical problems. If an underlying cause for pain is determined by medical examination, a specific treatment plan can be made to treat it.

Medications (narcotic or nonnarcotic) may be prescribed for moderate pain relief; for more powerful relief, muscle relaxants, tranquilizers, and possibly antidepressants may be prescribed. Intractable pain that does not respond to medication may warrant a nerve block. Back pain due to a disk problem is sometimes treated by surgically correcting the disk.

Chinese Treatment

Chinese medical experts, like their Western counterparts, strongly advise anyone experiencing pain to consult a professional to identify or rule out potential medical problems.

In cases of pain, it is especially beneficial to consult an M.D./acupuncturist (or an M.D. and an acupuncturist who can collaborate well). Many kinds of pain can be effectively relieved by acupuncture. Indeed, acupuncture is best known as a treatment for pain, and scientific studies have confirmed its ability to assist in the release of pain-killing endorphins (the body's natural mechanisms for controlling pain). As a result, many Western medical clinics or centers have a multidisciplinary approach to pain management that incorporates acupuncture.

For home treatment, see the section below that concerns the particular kind of pain involved:

For ankle pain, massage the following points, as appropriate:
- for pain at the top of the ankle: ST 41
- for pain deep inside the ankle: SP 5
- for pain on the outside of the ankle: BL 60
- for swelling around the anklebone on the inside of the leg: LR 3

For arm pain, massage the following points, as appropriate:
- for any arm pain: massage along the two sides of the lower back of the neck to stimulate nerves to the arm; also massage LI 9 as well as LI 4 (relieves pain and spasm; improves the flow of Qi and blood in the arm and fingers)
- for arm pain affecting the arm, elbow, and shoulder: LI 10 and LI 11
- for pain on the outer (little finger) side of the arm and hand: SI 3
- for pain on the back of the arm: TB 5

For back pain, consult with a doctor to make sure the pain is not related to a disk problem. In such cases it is not advisable to massage the back.

For elbow pain, massage the following points, as appropriate:
- for all elbow pain: LI 11
- for difficulty in raising the elbow: LI 5
- for pain on the outside of the elbow: SI 8

For finger pain, massage the following points, as appropriate:
- massage along the two sides of the spine from the lower neck to the upper back to stimulate the nerves to the finger
- LI 5
- the Ba Xie points: in the web between the fingers, closer toward the back of the hand
- for pain when bending fingers: TB 3

For hip pain, massage the following points, as appropriate:
- for any tender point in the hip area: massage along the two sides of the lower back to stimulate the lumbar nerves to the hip
- for sciatica and hip pain: GB 30
- for hip pain radiating to the groin: GB 29
- for difficulty in moving the hip and the knee: BL 40

For knee pain, massage the following points, as appropriate:
- for any knee pain: ST 35 and medial MN-LE 16 (the two "eyes" of the knee), SP 9, and ST 34
- for difficulty in extending the knee (by straightening the leg): massage along the two sides of the lower back to stimulate the lumbar nerves to the knee
- for difficulty in flexing the knee (by bending the leg): massage along the sides of the lower back to the sacral region above the tailbone to stimulate the nerves for flexing the knee

For shoulder pain, massage the following points, as appropriate:
- for any shoulder pain: massage along the sides of the lower cervical spine at the base of the neck to stimulate the nerves to the shoulders; LI 15 (improves the ability to raise the arm to the head) and LI 11
- for pain in the back of the shoulder or "frozen" shoulder: TB 14
- for pain in the shoulder blade (scapula): any tender point in the blade

For wrist pain, massage the following points, as appropriate:
- for pain on the side of the wrist below the thumb: LI 5
- for pain on the side of the wrist below the little finger: SI 4
- for swelling and general wrist pain: TB 4

Scars

Symptoms

Thickening of the skin, typically painful and red when forming; once formed, usually no longer painful (see below, "Description"), but maybe stiff-feeling.

Description

A scar is a segment of tissue that is no longer living—the aftereffect of a wound, cut, or a scrape. The depth of the scar indicates the seriousness of the damage. For example, a shallow scar from a cut or scrape probably does not sever any nerves, while a deep scar from abdominal surgery transects across nerves and blood vessels.

Scar tissue itself doesn't have nerve and blood supplies, and the surrounding nerves and blood vessels may be oddly reconfigured as a result of the original trauma and the scar formation. The scar tissue may stick to the surrounding healthy tissue so that it causes localized pain symptoms; for example, an abdominal scar attached to intestinal tissue may occasionally cause pain and even obstruction.

In Chinese medical theory, scars can have a significant effect on one's health. They represent potential Qi blocks, especially when they are raised, inflamed with redness, and/or uncomfortable or even painful when touched or massaged.

Deep scars, such as surgical ones, can obstruct Qi and blood flow in the immediate area or from one part of the body to another. The obstruction can be felt as pain, discomfort, a lack of energy, or even a sensation of weakness below the scar and hardness (or tightness) above it. For this reason, deep scars need to be treated by opening up the Qi flow. Acupuncture accomplishes this purpose with a treatment called "turtle technique": surrounding the scar with needles directed toward it.

Western Treatment

Steroids can be injected into scars to shrink them if they are big or unsightly. Scars with adhesions that cause symptoms may need to be removed by surgery or laser-cutting. Western medicine is usually not concerned about small, superficial scars.

Chinese Treatment

All scars regardless of size or depth can potentially block Qi flow and need to be treated. To help increase Qi input into the scarred area, do the following:

- Massage around the scar in a clockwise motion.
- Massage the Qi channel for the scarred area in the proper direction. When the scar is on the inside of the leg, massage the inside of the leg from the ankle toward the groin; when the scar is on the outside of the leg, massage the outside of the leg from the hip toward the ankle. Massage the outside of the arm from the fingers to the shoulder; massage the inside of the arm from the armpit to the fingers.

Seizure

Symptom

Spasm or involuntary jerking of one or more parts of the body, possibly accompanied by loss of consciousness and mental confusion.

Description

Seizures can vary from so-called focal seizures localized in one area of the body, such as the the neck, the arm, or the leg, to so-called grand mal seizures affecting the whole body. There is also petit mal seizure, which consists of a brief period—usually a few seconds—of apparent "absence" or daydreaming. Febrile seizures, which are benign seizures related to high fever, may occur in children between six months and five years of age, with a peak incident rate between nine and twenty months.

More than two-thirds of all seizure conditions begin in childhood. According to Western medicine, the causes of seizure depend on the age of onset. In the newborn period they include congenital malformations, insults to the brain (such as low oxygen or low blood sugar), and various metabolic disorders. In early childhood the causes include birth-related injuries, infections (such as meningitis or encephalitis), and trauma (such as a blow to the head). Another trigger may be the flashing lights of vivid graphics in video games. In adolescence and early adulthood the causes tend to be trauma, drugs, or hereditary predisposition, although there are also cases deemed idiopathic (of unknown cause). Among mature adults the most common causes are vascular disease, tumor, trauma, or withdrawal from drugs or alcohol.

Chinese medicine attributes seizure to a manifestation of "internal wind." Wind—whether internal (in the body) or external (in Nature)—has the characteristic of coming on suddenly and moving quickly. For internal wind this means rapid changes in physical symptoms and body-part locale. In severe instances internal wind can shake up the body just as an external wind shakes up a tree—causing a flailing of limbs and maybe even an "uprooting," which, in a body, translates into convulsions or even temporary limpness.

Among the causes of such internal wind disturbances are acute illnesses with fever, especially among children under six years old, and windborne infections, which are analogous to the Western concept of infectious diseases such as meningitis and encephalitis. Wind is associated with the Liver, which is an organ of metabolism, so any injury of the Liver from whatever cause—drugs, alcohol, infections, or trauma—can result in internal wind. This relates to the Western notion of metabolic causes of seizure. Head trauma can cause seizure by creating a blood stasis (or pool) that blocks Qi and blood movement inside the brain. A deficiency in Kidney Essence (hereditary) also can lead to seizure.

Chinese medicine also defines an injury to the digestive system as a possible cause of seizure. Spleen Qi can be weakened by previous episodes of severe, gastrointestinal illnesses or by excessive intake of phlegm-producing foods. The result is heat that moves upward, blocking energy channels and stirring up Liver wind. In such cases the person's skin may appear sallow and, during the seizure, there may be frothing in the mouth or gurgling in the throat. Petit mal seizures or "staring spells" are often associated with Spleen Qi deficiency.

Western Treatment

During a seizure itself, it's important to make sure the person does not injure himself or herself, so remove any potentially dangerous objects from the vicinity, and do what you can to cushion possible trauma spots or divert the person away from them. As a general rule, do not hold fast to the arms or the legs or put hard objects in the mouth. Instead, allow the seizure to run its course and come to a stop by itself. In a hospital context, suppositories or intravenous medications can be given to stop the seizure.

For treatment of the seizure, consult a professional to find the cause, and then follow the appropriate course of action. Anticonvulsant medications such as phenobarbitol, Dilantin, or valproic acid may be used singly or in combination. The dosage of such medications must be monitored very closely because there may be significant side effects. Home treatment includes decreased use of alcohol and drugs; a well-balanced diet; and good eating habits (regular meals, eaten slowly with no distraction).

Chinese Treatment

During a seizure, follow the same guidelines given under "Western Treatment" above. In addition, two points may be "hard-massaged" by pinching them or pressing them hard with the nails: DU 26 (if there's no violent jerking of the head and it's accessible) and KI 1 (if there's no violent jerking of the legs and it's accessible).

To treat the seizure, consult a doctor. Acupuncture can be very helpful in treating seizure and in weaning a person to a smaller dose of seizure medication. (*Note:* Do not try this tapering-off process without close monitoring by a M.D.-acupuncturist or a M.D. and an acupuncturist working in close cooperation.)

Also do the following:

- Massage LI 4, P 6, LR 3, GB 34, KI 1, and SP 6.
- To clear heat, massage LI 11.
- To clear brain orifices, massage DU 14, and DU 20.
- For seizure associated with infection, massage LI 4, LI 11, and DU 14.
- For seizure with gurgling, massage CV 22 and ST 40.
- For head trauma, to decrease blood stasis, massage LR 2, LR 3, and BL 17.
- Decrease intake of phlegm-producing foods, alcohol, and anything injurious to the Liver.

Sighing, Excessive or Chronic

Symptoms

Audible breathing, usually on expiration.

Description

In Western medicine, sighing is generally due to an underlying emotional problem.

Chinese medicine attributes sighing to a Qi imbalance that may have a physical or an emotional cause. Qi accumulates in the chest and creates pressure there, which is expelled through hard breathing. In most cases the Qi imbalance originates in the Spleen channel, and it also can affect the Liver and Heart channels in their Five-Element Relationship.

Western Treatment

If the underlying emotional problem is deemed significant, it may be treated with medication or psychotherapy. Otherwise no treatment is offered to alleviate the sighing itself.

Chinese Treatment

To open the chest, move Qi, and calm the spirit, Chinese medical experts recommend the steps listed below. If the condition persists, the person needs to consult with a professional to evaluate the underlying cause or causes of sighing.

- Massage SP 1, SP 15, P 6, HT 7, GB 34, LR 3, and CV 15.
- If sadness is experienced along with sighing, massage GB 24.
- Do calming exercises (see chapter 5).
- Review *Emotional Problems* in this guide to determine if any of the descriptions fit the situation. If so, follow the appropriate guidelines.

Snoring

Symptoms

Audible, often ragged breathing, sometimes accompanied by short stopping or "skipping" of breath (apnea).

Description

Western medicine usually attributes snoring to an anatomical cause—often a tonsil enlargement that obstructs the air passage. In Chinese medical terms, snoring results from a disturbance in the flow of Qi. When the Qi that should flow downward does not, it "rebels" upward at night, causing noisy breathing. Excess phlegm is frequently the source of the Qi flow imbalance.

Western Treatment

Surgery to relieve any anatomical obstruction; otherwise, changing the sleeping position, either voluntarily, or when nudged by a partner, or when signaled by one of various over-the-counter devices; or wearing an over-the-counter tape on the nose to widen or reform the nasal passages.

Chinese Treatment

Before going to bed, do the following:
- Massage the lateral/outer surface of each leg downward (fifty strokes for each leg, which takes one to two minutes).
- Massage the E micromeridian on the lateral surface on the palm side of the fifth finger, from the palm toward the tip (fifty strokes).
- Massage ST 40 and P 6.

Also avoid phlegm-producing foods.

Sore Throat, Pharyngitis or Tonsillitis

Symptoms

Soreness of throat, possibly accompanied by any of the following: redness, fever, pus, red dots on the palate, dryness, or coughing.

Description

From a Western perspective, the origin of a sore throat is a viral or bacterial infection, the most common bacterium being the streptococcus, which causes strep throat. Any case of sore throat can be further described as either sudden/acute or chronic/recurrent.

In general, the viral sore throat is usually milder, and often unaccompanied by other symptoms, such as fever or pus. A bacterial or strep throat more commonly produces one or more of these symptoms and, possibly, red dots on the palate. It is also

255

frequently part of a cluster of other respiratory problems—for example, dryness or coughing. A chronic/recurrent sore throat may be caused by a debilitated physical state that predisposes the person to recurrent infections or by repeated exposure to a strep carrier.

In Chinese medicine, an acute/sudden sore throat is attributed to an invasion by external wind-heat. A chronic/recurrent case points to an internal imbalance, usually a state of Yin deficiency.

Western Treatment

A professional throat culture is advised to determine whether the problem is strep throat. If so, it is generally treated with antibiotics to avoid the risk of developing rheumatic fever . If it's not strep, it usually can be treated with throat lozenges and gargles for relief of symptoms. Analgesics such as Tylenol can be taken to relieve pain.

Chinese Treatment

- For acute/sudden sore throat: Massage LI 4, LI 11, ST 44, LU 11, CV 22, and DU 14. Also eat cooling and neutral foods.
- For chronic/recurrent sore throat: In addition to the above-listed points, massage KI 3 and KI 6 to tonify the Kidney. Also eat foods that tonify the Kidney.

Stuttering

Symptoms

Involuntary delay or rapid repetition of speech.

Description

Stuttering is normal in the speech development of children under age four and usually goes away by age six. When stuttering persists to, or occurs at, a later age, Western medicine considers it a "habit disorder" rather than a nerve dysfunction. In some cases there may be a psychological factor—for example, stuttering due to emotional stress or to the desire for attention or sympathy.

The Chinese medical explanation correlates to the Western one. In Chinese terms, the Heart is the seat of the Mind (the center of emotions) and controls speech (or, as the Chinese put it, "the Heart opens into the tongue"). Therefore, stuttering in young children is considered a normal possible stumbling block in their maturation process—speech control developing along with emotional control. Stuttering at a later age is attributed to problems in Heart Qi.

Western Treatment

In the case of a child under age six, it is important for listeners to understand that stuttering is a normal part of his or her development and not to call attention to it. For stuttering at a later age, speech therapy is advisable. Among the techniques used in such therapy are breath control exercises and speech-pacing with the help of miniaturized metronomes. If a psychological factor is suspected, some form of psychotherapy also may be prescribed.

Chinese Treatment

In addition to the Western recommendations, massage HT 5.

Thrush

Symptoms

White patches or scattered white spots, with or without red borders, inside the mouth, possibly accompanied by fever, flushed face, red lips, restlessness, pale complexion, or warm palms.

Description

In Western medicine, the cause of oral thrush is a fungal (candida) infection. It often occurs in infants and young children, especially during or after antibiotic treatment. In Chinese medicine, thrush is attributed to a variety of causes, ranging from excess heat within the body to improper diet.

Western Treatment

Oral Nystatin or Gentian Violet swabbed onto the walls of the mouth.

Chinese Treatment
- Massage LI 11 to clear heat
- Massage ST 40, and CV 23
- Massage the hand microsystem mapping of the face, located on the distal phalange of the third finger
- Massage the hand F micromeridian, in the middle of the palm side of the fifth finger, massage from the tip toward the palm
- Avoid excess intake of hot foods.

Toothache

Symptoms

Dull or sharp pain in a tooth and/or the gum, possibly accompanied by throbbing, swelling, palpitations, thirst, or halitosis ("bad breath").

Description

A toothache may be a secondary indication of tooth decay (dental caries) or gum disease, so it is important to consult a dentist as soon as possible. *Note:* Ask your dentist about the safety of using various cavity-filling substances (amalgams) for dental caries. Do your own, independent research on the subject as well. Many practitioners of complementary medicine believe that amalgams, which are difficult to remove entirely from the body, can cause various kinds of health problems.

If the toothache is accompanied by flu symptoms such as fever or chills, the probable cause is a viral or bacterial infection that needs additional treatment as influenza.

Chinese medicine posits that Qi disturbance can contribute to the formation of dental caries and gum disease. Excessive heat in the Stomach channel affects the upper gum. Excessive heat in the Large Intestine affects the lower gum. In addition or alternatively, there may be a deficiency in the Kidney channel causing the tooth to ache. If so, the toothache often gets worse at bedtime.

Western Treatment

Pain medications for symptomatic relief. People with a toothache are advised to see a dentist as soon as possible.

Chinese treatment:
- For any toothache, massage LI 4.
- For an ache in an upper tooth, also massage ST 7.
- For an ache in a lower tooth, also massage ST 6.
- For a toothache that gets worse at night, also massage KI 3.

Glossary

biopsychotype   The five different physical and emotional types of human beings classified according to the Five Elements.

Corporeal Soul   The Soul of our body, residing in the Lung. It comes to us at birth and dies with us.

destructive cycle   Refers to the "controlling" or "destructive" relationship of one element with another element.

Essence *(Jing)*   A powerful substance that carries genetic information and influences our development, sexual functioning, and aging. It is associated with the Kidney.

Ethereal Soul   The Soul of the mind, residing in Liver Yin. It comes to us at birth and returns to the Soul World upon our death. It brings images from the Soul World.

Five Elements   Water, Wood, Fire, Earth, and Metal; corresponding elements in human beings and Nature; foods, organ systems, and biopsychotypes are classified according to these elements.

macrocosm   A larger pattern that is reflected by a smaller one. In Chinese medicine, Nature is the macrocosm reflected in each human being.

microcosm   A smaller pattern that reflects a larger one. In Chinese medicine, a human being is a microcosm of Nature.

microsystem   Miniature mappings of the whole human body or Qi system upon a small area of the body; examples of microsystems: ears, hands, abdomen, feet, and tongue.

Mind   Refers to the intellectual and mental-emotional aspects of our being and is connected to the human spirit via the Ethereal Soul.

nurturing cycle   Refers to the Five-Element relationship when an Element nurtures the next element in the cycle.

Qi   The vital energy that circulates within the human body in channels called meridians. It is also part of the blood and the organs. In addition, it is a universal energy that connects all living things on Earth. It is Yang as compared to Blood, Fluid, and Essence, which are Yin.

Soul   The spirit of human beings. There are two Souls: the Ethereal Soul and the Corporeal Soul.

Three Treasures of Life   Refers to Qi, mind, and Essence. Collectively these constitute the physical and the emotional parts of human beings and are intimately related to the spiritual parts: the Ethereal Soul and the Corporeal Soul.

Yang   The interdependent, mutually inclusive opposite of Yin. The balance of Yin-Yang is the basis of all natural phenomena and human processes.

Yin   The interdependent, mutually inclusive opposite of Yang. The balance of Yin-Yang is the basis of all natural phenomena and human processes.

A Word about Herbs

In recent years Chinese herbs have become increasingly popular as more Westerners have been turning to Chinese medicine. Although a few herbs, such as ginseng, are especially well known, it is easy to find a variety of herbs in herbal stores, health food stores, and even some grocery stores. Herbs have very powerful medicinal effects, however, and should not be used indiscriminately. I'm going to give you some basic facts about Chinese herbs so you can have a better understanding of what they are and how they work. My advice is to consult a herbalist before using herbs so that you consume only the ones that are appropriate for you.

The healing effects of Chinese herbs depend on the time and the place of harvest, their taste, their thermoregulatory (temperature regulation) properties, the different Qi channels they enter, and the overall effect on the human body.

In ancient times, herbs were carefully harvested in their natural environment at key times of the day or season that had the optimal soil, moisture, or sunlight. For example, one herb may be harvested by the riverbed, early in the morning, in late summer; while another one is harvested by the mountainside, in the late afternoon, in autumn. To this day, people in different parts of China cultivate different herbs according to the local climate and topography. Herbs also continue to be harvested when the healing ingredients are most plentiful. For example, some of the leaves are harvested in late summer, some flowers in their budding stage, some roots when they are young and tender.

Herbs are classified according to their taste: sweet, bitter, sour, salty, pungent or bland. They are also classified according to what they do to the temperature of the body: hot, warm, neutral, cool, or cold. These properties are discussed in chapter 4 in terms of food and beverages. Because herbs are foods, it is no surprise that they have the same properties. It also follows that since different flavors of food affect different organs, so do different flavors of herbs. Herbs are further classified according to their general impact throughout the body—for example, they may basically clear heat, transform phlegm, tonify Qi, tonify blood, or calm the spirit.

Let's use ginseng as an example. Ginseng is a root that comes in many varieties. The most effective grows in the wild and is called wild mountain root. Most of the ginseng sold in the world today (including in the United States and China) is cultivated, not wild. Ginseng has a sweet and mildly bitter taste. It also has slightly warming properties. It preferentially enters the Spleen/Pancreas and Lung channels. Ginseng is very good as an overall Qi tonic—and especially potent as a tonic for the Lung and the Spleen. However, it should not be used by someone who is Yin-deficient with heat symptoms, or who has a condition such as high blood pressure, headache, or heart palpitations.

The classic way of taking herbs is to make a tea concoction out of a combination of raw herbs. The raw herbs need to be processed in different ways to maximize their healing effects—

for example, by removing the outer layer that has no medicinal value and by slicing or grinding the herb to increase its surface area.

Specific herbs are combined to maximize healing effects and to minimize side effects. The herb is ranked according to its importance in the formula. The "emperor" herb is the most important herb that exerts the principal effect, and other herbs, such as "minister," "helper," or "servant" herbs, perform various supportive functions. One or two herbs are also added to the combination to minimize side effects.

Raw herbal tea is the most powerful form of herbal medication. However, most of us find it inconvenient to take hours to make the tea. Besides, it usually winds up having a strong smell and an unpleasant taste. We usually prefer the Western-style pill or powder form of the herb. While some herbalists still prepare herbs in the traditional way as teas, the majority of herbalists settle for the modern pill or powder preparation to have better patient compliance.

Herbs are vastly different from Western medications in these major areas:

1. Herbs are foods. The vast majority of herbs are plants, with a small variety of herbs coming from animal parts.
2. Herbs are all-natural substances, while Western medications are usually synthetic compounds made by pharmaceutical companies.
3. Herbs are mild and usually need to be taken for a relatively lengthy period of time before they show effect. Medications are very powerful and can show effects usually within minutes or hours.
4. Herbal preparations include herbs to counteract or to soften the side effects of the "emperor" herb. Medications generally do not contain such buffering agents.
5. Herbs can tonify the body as a whole, while medications

usually treat only symptoms and do not have an overall strengthening purpose.

• Herbs are used to bring the body into balance. Medications are usually used to treat symptoms.

Chinese medicine considers Western medications to be very powerful substances that can produce wonderful results fairly quickly but tend to weaken the body if they're taken over a long period of time. Although some medications were originally extracted from natural substances (the most well-known example is penicillin taken from mold), almost all of them are synthesized in laboratories. There is a big difference between ingesting the herb as a whole and ingesting just the active chemical ingredients in manufactured form.

For example, the ephedra herb has many other ingredients that help temper its effects, and it is usually taken with other herbs to make it gentler on the human constitution. The chemical ingredient ephedrine used to treat asthma is so powerful by itself that it has the effect of giving the body a jolt. There are times when we need that kind of stimulus, such as when an infection needs to be cleared up quickly. In chronic situations, however, it is difficult for the body to handle such a powerful impact regularly.

Whatever you decide to do regarding herbal medication, it won't take the place of following the dietary, exercise, and treatment guidelines recommended in this book. Herbs can, however, provide you with another great way of caring for yourself and your loved ones. Good luck to you in your future explorations of this realm of Chinese medicine.

Overcoming the Side Effects of Western Medications

Both Western and Chinese medicine share the common goal of healing. Their treatment approaches, however, are different, especially in the preparation and administration of medications.

Chinese medications are derived mainly from whole plants that are cooked slowly so their Qi and thermoregulatory properties are preserved. The effect of taking them is natural and mild. Western medications are synthesized in laboratories so that only active molecules are incorporated into the final product. The result is a very potent chemical medication that can act as a shock to our physical constitution.

There are times when a fast-acting, powerful jolt is necessary to combat a particularly dangerous or vigorous disease. A classic example is the knockout punch of antibiotics, which have saved millions of lives and have radically decreased our vulnerability to bacterial infections that might otherwise overwhelm our immune system. However, the disadvantages of using chemical medications are:

- They are not natural to, nor can they tonify, our body systems because they do not contain Qi.
- Powerful side effects can cause diseases by themselves. In fact, they're currently responsible for 10 percent of hospital admissions.
- An overprescription or abuse of medications (often unintentional) can result in the emergence of new or more difficult-to-treat conditions, as in the case of antibiotics, which have resulted in the emergence of stronger strains of bacteria that are drug-resistant.

Nevertheless, chemical medications of all kinds are here to stay. One of the best integrations of Western and Chinese medicine involves using both simultaneously to derive more health benefits and to avoid, minimize, or recover more effectively from any chemical-related side effects. In China and other Asian countries, hospital patients often receive chemical medications through one intravenous (IV) line and, at the same time, herbal solutions through another.

This appendix describes the possible side effects of the three most widely used categories of chemical medications and tells you how to avoid or treat these effects with simple Chinese medical treatments.

First, here are guidelines that can help you devise your own, more customized and comprehensive East-West treatment plan for the medication or medications you are taking:

- From all the information about side effects that accompanies your medication or medications—including labels on the container, package inserts, and pharmacy printouts—determine whether each side effect is Yin or Yang in nature, using the guidelines in chapter 2. Then group all the Yin effects together (assuming there are any) and all the Yang effects together (again, assuming there are any). If the group of Yin entries is bigger, follow guidelines in this book for treating a Yin deficiency, and vice versa.

The key is to look for a *group* of side effects that all fall into a Yin or a Yang category. For example, the side effect of a dry mouth alone does not indicate that the medication or medications may cause a Yin (fluid) deficiency. However, if there's a group of Yin-related side effects such as a dry mouth, dry skin, and constipation, the risk of a Yin deficiency is very likely.

- Because no chemical medication tonifies an organ system, you should use Chinese medicine to do so. Consult the appropriate guidelines in this book for tonifying the organ system or systems involved in the illness.
- General Qi tonifying is advisable during any kind of illness and can be especially beneficial whenever you're taking chemical medications. Therefore, do more breathing, meditation, movement, and singing exercises (see chapter 5).
- Because the majority of chemical medications can cause digestive symptoms and are metabolized by the liver, it's a good idea to follow the guidelines in this book for tonifying your Stomach, Spleen/Pancreas, and Liver.
- To counteract cold effects, massage KI 3 and KI 7.

Listed below are recommendations for avoiding or treating side effects relating to three major kinds of Western medications: antibiotics, tricyclic antidepressants, and steroids.

Antibiotics

All antibiotics are anti-inflammatory. In Chinese medical terms, it means that they are Cold in Nature (inflammation being Hot) and can do everything that Cold foods do, such as slowing Qi flow.

In addition, antibiotics harm normal bacteria in the Stomach, thereby injuring Stomach Yin, and most can cause hypersensitive reactions such as rashes (urticaria), which are associated in Chinese medicine with blood heat and a Liver Yin deficiency.

To counteract any or all of these negative effects while you're taking antibiotics, do the following:

- Avoid excess Hot or Cold foods, and increase intake of Warm foods and liquids (e.g., chicken soup).
- Tonify Stomach Yin by massaging these points: CV 12, ST 36, SP 6, and SP 3.
- Tonify Liver Yin by massaging these points: KI 6, LR 8, and LR 3.

Tricyclic Antidepressants

The precise mechanism of tricyclic antidepressants—which include imipramine (Tofranil), amitriptyline (Norpramin), and nortriptyline (Aventyl)—is not known, although there is evidence that such drugs lead to an increase of neurotransmitters in the brain. In Western medicine, depression is attributed to a deficiency of neurotransmitters.

Among the possible negative side effects of tricyclic antidepressants are low blood pressure (hypotension), heart palpitations, irregular heartbeat (arrhythmia), insomnia, agitation, and restlessness.

From a Chinese medical standpoint, these side effects are due to a scattering of Yang from the Kidney and the blood, and a Qi deficiency in the Heart. Therefore it is important to tonify the Heart Yin, the Heart Qi, and Kidney Yang by doing the following things:

- Avoid bitter foods and cut down on excessively salty foods.
- Massage the upper back in a clockwise fashion and these points: CV 6, CV 17, KI 3, KI 6, KI 7, and P 6.

Steroids

Prolonged use of steroids can have profound effects all over the body, including pituitary and other glandular problems, muscle weakness, bone damage (osteoporosis), ulcers, rashes, the thinning of the skin, hormone imbalances, and increased eye pressure, increased hair growth (hirsutism).

From a Chinese medical standpoint, steroids are Essence-like substances capable of causing major changes in growth, body development, sexual function, and aging. The result of such changes is a depletion of the body's own hard-to-regenerate natural Essence, associated with Kidney Yin. Kidney Qi and Kidney Yang are similarly depleted.

Here are recommendations for avoiding or treating these side effects:

- Avoid excessive intake of sweet foods or foods high in protein (the latter increase the load on the Kidney). Also avoid alcohol, coffee, tobacco, and hard drugs. Men should decrease their frequency of ejaculation (men lose Essence in their semen).
- Increase intake of vitamins and foods that are nurturing for Essence, such as microalgae, vitamin A, vitamin B12, and organic animal organs such as kidneys and livers; honeybee products such as royal jelly and bee pollen; millet; wheat; black sesame seeds; black soybeans; chestnuts; raspberries; strawberries; and walnuts.
- Avoid stress and overwork.

- To help preserve Essence, do meditation and movement exercises (see chapter 5).
- To nourish the Kidney and Essence, massage CV 4, KI 1, KI 3, KI 6, KI 7, and KI 9.

The Acupressure Points and Diagrams of the Body Channels

General information about acupressure points:

1. Acupressure points usually are located between muscles, in spots that feel like a "dip" or a "hollow spot," so that when you press on an acupressure point, your finger feels as if it is "falling into a hole." Many of the points will feel tender, which is an indication that something is wrong there and needs to be treated.

2. The measurements are taken as the width of one "finger-breadth" (abbreviated FB), which is the measurement of the width of the thumb. The width is taken from the *person's* thumb. If you are massaging a child or a very thin or overweight person, you need to measure the width of that person's thumb and *approximate* it to your fingers. You do not need to worry about exact precision, since your finger will mostly likely sense the point as it "falls into the hole"; as you

massage, you would cover a much bigger spot than would an acupuncture needle.

3. There are many different ways to combine points for a given disorder. The points in this book are chosen for two reasons: (1) they are major points or "big points" that can exert a powerful effect and (2) they are easy to locate.

The points are illustrated both as channels (so you have an overall picture for the entire channel) and as points grouped according to their locations on the body. Only the points mentioned in this book are illustrated. The channels are listed in the classic sequence of showing Yin-Yang coupling and principal meridian connections. Most books on acupuncture/acupressure list the channels and points in this sequence.

The micromeridians are located on the hands. The individual channels that are used in this book are located on the fourth and fifth fingers, and designated according to Dr. Yoo's letter system. The diagram shows the direct mapping of the body onto the hands.

A word of clarification of the terms "inside" and "outside":

- inside of arm: the palmar side
- outside of arm: the side of the back of the hand
- inside of leg: facing the midline of the body
- outside of leg: facing outside

Body Points

Lung

LU 5   *Location:* On the inside crease of the elbow. Roll your thumb along the elbow from the outside (the back side of the thumb) toward the inside (the palm side), you'll come to a "hollow." If you move your thumb farther, you'll touch a tendon. This point is in the hollow space before the tendon.

Function: This is the Water point on the Lung channel and is an important point for clearing "heat" or infections in the Lungs.

LU 7 *Location:* Locate the "dent" below your thumb on the wrist, the classic "anatomic snuff box." Slide your finger across the forearm bone, the radius, and you'll come to a "dent" inside the radius about 1½ FB (thumb-width distance) from the snuff box.

Function: This is a major point on the Lung channel and is used for a variety of Lung disorders, including expelling wind and making Lung Qi move in the right direction downward.

LU 9 *Location:* At the wrist below the thumb, roll your finger from the outside toward the middle of the palmar side; the first hollow you feel is LU 9.

Function: This the most important point for tonifying or strengthening the Lung.

LU 10 *Location:* About the middle of the "pad" below the thumb—the thenar eminence.

Function: This is the fire point on the Lung channel. Sedating it: when it is massaged counterclockwise, (i.e., sedated), heat in the Lung channel is decreased

Large Intestine

LI 4 *Location:* It is located in the web space on the back of the hand between the thumb and index (second) finger, but closer to the index finger. It is often sore.

Functions: This is one of the most important points in the body. It ranks on a par with LR 3 for its powerful and global influences of the whole body. It is used in many disorders, including any problems with the face and head; regulating Defensive Qi that protects us against adverse external factors; and restoring Yang. Because of its power, massage with caution, especially with children, who may not be able to handle a strong stimulus.

LI 5   *Location:* Keep your thumb straight and feel the "hollow" on the side of the wrist below the thumb—the anatomical "snuff box."

Functions: This point helps raise the elbow as well as decrease pain in wrist and fingers.

LI 9   *Location:* Draw an imaginary line from LI 5 to LI 11. LI 9 is 3 FB below LI 11 on that line.

Function: This point helps with any pain of the arms.

LI 10   *Location:* This point is between LI 9 and LI 11: 2 FB below LI 11, 1 FB above LI 9.

Functions: This point is the "Arm Three Mile" point, which is used to treat pain in the shoulder, elbow, arm, and hands.

LI 11   *Location:* Bend your elbow. Feel the hollow right at the end of the elbow crease.

Functions: This is a major point for clearing heat from anywhere in the body. It can cool heat from Blood, and regulate Qi and Blood. It is the Earth point on the Large Intestine Channel, and can be used to activate Qi flow in the meridian.

LI 15   *Location:* Raise your arm to the side, up to shoulder height. Feel the hollow just in front (toward the chest side) of the top of the shoulder. In most people you can actually see a dimple or a depression there.

Functions: This is a very good point for treating shoulder pain, stiffness, weakness, or difficulty in raising the arm. It is usually massaged along with TB 14 to increase effectiveness.

LI 16 *Location:* On the upper back of the shoulder, move your finger from the tip of the shoulder toward the neck; you'll feel a hollow at the point where the clavicle forms a fork with the shoulder blade.

Function: This is a good point for treating shoulder problems.

LI 20 *Location:* In the groove next to the nose, at the same level as the middle of the nostrils.

Functions: This is a good point for opening up the nasal passages and getting rid of upper airway infections and congestion.

Stomach

ST 4 *Location:* Next to the corners of the mouth, less than half a FB's width.

Function: This is a good point for treating drooling and for numbness of the mouth and the face.

ST 6 *Location:* Locate the point by first clenching your teeth, and feel the tightened muscle below the ear and slightly above the angle of the jaw. After finding the point, unclench your teeth and massage the point with the muscle relaxed.

Function: A good point for pain in lower teeth.

ST 7 *Location:* Locate the point by first opening your mouth and feel the tight muscle in front of the ear; this muscle disappears and becomes a "hollow point" when the mouth is closed.

Function: A good point for pain in upper teeth.

ST 25 *Location:* Two FB next to the navel on both sides.

Functions: A big point for problems of the Large Intestine. Can also be used to regulate the Spleen and the Stomach.

ST 29   *Location:* Four FB below the the belly button, 2 FB to the side from the midline, at same level as CV 3.

        Function: This point helps with menstruation and warms the womb.

ST 30   *Location:* Right above the top border of the pubis, 2 FB to the side of the midline on both sides.

        Functions: A good point for regulating Qi in the Lower Burner and for menstrual problems.

ST 34   *Location:* Two FB above the outside border of the patella, the kneecap.

        Function: A very good point for treatment or knee problems.

ST 35   *Location:* The two "dents" below the kneecap, often called the "eyes" of the knee.

        Function: Good for treating any knee problems.

ST 36   *Location:* 3 FB below ST 35, the "eye" of the knee, on the outside border of the tibia, the big bone of the lower leg.

        Function: This is the famous "Leg Three Mile" Point— a very major point, also known as the Master of Immunity Point. This point is said to be able to treat anything. It can strengthen the immune system, give an energy boost, and can calm the mind. It is useful for many digestive disorders.

ST 40   *Location:* Roughly halfway between the anklebone and the bottom of the kneecap, 2 FB lateral to or one muscle mass on the outside of the front border of the tibia.

        Function: A major point for treating phlegm, which is associated with cough and wheezing in Western medicine but also can be associated with some pain conditions in Chinese medicine.

ST 41   *Location:* Middle of the top of the ankle; feels like a "hole."

       Functions: This can be a local point for pain of the ankle, or a distal point for belching.

ST 43   *Location:* On the top of the foot, in the web space between the second and third toes, about 1½ FB from the edge of the web, where ST 44 is located.

       Function: This is a useful point for treating edema and abdominal pain. It is the Wood point on the Earth Stomach channel and is good for decreasing excess Yang symptoms. Used together with ST 44 for sedation.

ST 44   *Location:* On the top of the foot, just inside the edge of the web between the second and the third toes.

       Function: Water point on the Stomach channel. Can be used to clear heat, and also used with ST 43 to calm the mind.

ST 45   *Location:* Approximately 0.1 inch from the outside corner of the second toenail.

       Function: The last point on the ST channel, a good distal point to treat gastritis and nervous stomach.

Spleen

SP 1   *Location:* On top of the tip of the big toe, right under the inside, lower border of the nail.

      Function: A strong point to stop bleeding.

SP 2   *Location:* Feel along the side of the big toe from SP 1, right before the "bump" where the big toe joins the foot.

      Function: It is good for treating "excess dampness," which manifests as edema or swelling in the limbs.

SP 3   *Location:* On the side of the foot below the prominent bone of the big toe.

       Function: A good point for activating Spleen energy.

SP 4   *Location:* First locate SP 3, then slide your finger along the side of the foot toward the ankle. This point is located right in front of the next bone.

       Function: This is a good point for menstrual problems and for abdominal pain.

SP 5   *Location:* This point is on the inside of the foot, right below the front border of the anklebone.

       Function: This is a useful point for treating pain on the inside of the ankle.

SP 6   *Location:* On the inside of the leg, about 3 FB above the inside ankle. Put your finger on top of the edge of the ankle and slide upward along the inside of the tibia and you'll come to a hollow. It is usually tender, especially in women.

       Function: This is the most important Yin point in the body. It is the crossing of the three Yin channels of the leg: Liver, Spleen, Kidney. It can be used for overall tonification or strengthening of Qi, Blood, and Yin. It strengthens the three Yin channels, regulates menstruation, and can calm the spirit.

SP 9   *Location:* On the inside of the leg, feel the "knob" (the top part of the tibia) next to the lower border of the kneecap, and go directly under the "knob." Usually it is tender in women.

       Function: It is the Water point on the Spleen channel and can be used to treat abdominal edema and swelling of the lower legs. It is also used as a local point for knee problems.

SP 10   *Location:* Put your finger 2 FB above the top of the kneecap and slide it toward the inside of the leg. You'll feel a tender hollow on the bulge of the muscle.

       Function: This point is good for menstrual problems and skin disorders such as urticaria and eczema.

SP 15   *Location:* At the level of the navel 4 FB from the midline on both sides.

       Function: This is a good point for moving Qi and regulating the intestines, for lower abdominal pain.

Heart

HT 5   *Location:* On the palm side of the wrist, 1 FB from the wrist on the fifth (little)-finger side.

       Function: Good for voice or speaking problems such as stuttering.

HT 7   *Location:* On the palm side, fifth (little)-finger side of the wrist, roll your finger from the side of the wrist toward the middle. You'll feel a "cord," which is a tendon; this point is right next to the cord in a hollow space.

       Function: This is a very important point for calming the excess symptoms of the Heart and for insomnia.

HT 8   *Location:* On the palm in a "dent" below the junction between fourth finger and the fifth (little) finger. If you make a fist, this point is where the tip of the little finger touches the palm.

       Function: The fire point on the Heart (fire) channel, it is a strong point to calm the mind and decrease palpitations.

Small Intestine

SI 1   *Location:* On the back of the hand, right on the outside of the lower border of the fifth fingernail.

Function: This is a good point for reviving consciousness.

SI 3   *Location:* When you make a loose fist, you'll see the crease of the hand fold into a bulging point on the side of the hand. SI 3 is located right under the bulge in a hollow space.

Function: This is a very good point for treating pain along the side of the arm, neck, and upper back. It also can influence the Governing channel, the major Yang channel located along the spine in the back.

SI 4   *Location:* On the side of the hand below the little finger, in a "dent" between the hand and the wrist.

Function: Good local point for wrist pain on that side of the hand.

SI 8   *Location:* With the elbow bent, this point is in the dent between two bony points on the tip of the elbow.

Function: This is a good point for treating pain of the elbow.

SI 19   *Location:* This point is best located with the mouth open. Feel the "hollow" in front of the ear.

Function: This is one of three points for treating ear problems such as ear infections: TB 21, GB 2, SI 19.

Bladder

BL 1   *Location:* Right above the top of the inside corner of the eye.

Function: This point is connected with channels that influence opening and closing of the eyes and therefore can be used to treat insomnia and drowsiness. It is also a good point for any eye conditions.

BL 13, 14, 15, 18, 19, 20, 21, 22, 23, 25, 27, and 28. These will be discussed together as the Back Shu or Transporting Points for the Organs. These points are directly connected to their respective organs and can be used to tonify (strengthen) the organs. The exact locations of points are difficult to know, especially in overweight individuals. However, for purposes of massage, you can just massage in the general area of the points. Better still, you can just massage the upper back for Lung and Heart, the middle back area for the Liver and digestive system, and the lower back for Kidney, Large Intestine, Small Intestine, and Bladder. I'll give a description for the precise locations for those interested readers or for readers who have had some experience doing acupressure.

Landmark location for BL 13–15: Run your finger down the neck along the midline. You will feel two bony "knobs" that stick out at the base of the neck. Put one thumb on one of the "knobs" and another thumb on the second "knob." Ask the person to turn his or her head from side to side. The one that moves is C 7, the last cervical vertebra. The "knob" that doesn't move is T 1, the first thoracic vertebra. Now you can start counting as you move your hand down the spine. The thoracic numbers go up as you move downward. The Bladder channel is located 1 1/2 FB from the midline on both sides on the highest point of the paraspinus muscles (the muscles along the sides of the spine).

Landmark location for BL 22–28: Feel for the top of the hipbone in the back. Go across to the midline. That is L 4, Lumbar 4, which corresponds to BL 25. Go up two spaces and you'll come to L 2, for BL 23; go up another space to L 1, for BL 22. Go down from BL 25 and you'll feel a hollow, a small opening in the sacral bone. That is the location for BL 27. BL 28 is located on the next hollow down from BL 27.

Bladder Channel Points

Transporting Points	Organ	Location	Spirit	Outer BL
BL 13	Lung 1	1½–FB next to T 3	Corporeal Soul	BL 42
BL 14	Master of Heart	T 4		
BL 15	Heart	T 5	Shen	BL 44
BL 18	Liver	T 9 (skips down from T 8)	Ethereal Soul	BL 47
BL 19	Gallbladder	T 10		
BL 20	Spleen	T 11	Thought	BL 49
BL 21	Stomach	T 12		
BL 22	Triple Burner	L 1		
BL 23	Kidney	L 2	Will	BL 52
BL 25	Large Intestine	L 4		
BL 27	Small Intestine	S 1		
BL 28	Bladder	S 2		

The outer Bladder lines are located 1½ FB from the inner Bladder lines and have five major points with spiritual values and are located in the same horizontal line next to the corresponding organ points.

BL 40 *Location:* Locate this point by slightly bending the knee; feel the "hollow" in the middle of the back of the knee.

Functions: This point has many functions but is good for treating back pain, knee pain, and hip pain.

BL 42 Corporeal Soul—next to Lung Shu BL 13

BL 44 Shen—next to Heart Shu BL 15

BL 47 Ethereal Soul—next to Liver Shu BL 18

BL 49 Thought—next to Spleen Shu BL 19

BL 52 Will—next to Kidney Shu BL 23

BL 57 *Location:* Come up the Achilles tendon until you come to a hollow between two muscles.

Function: Relaxes tendons and muscles to relieve pain in the lower leg.

BL 60 *Location:* On the outside of the foot, in the "dent" between the anklebone and the Achilles tendon.

Function: This point can be used to treat pain on the outside of the ankle.

BL 62 *Location:* This point is located directly below the outside anklebone.

Function: A good point for relieving pain, for opening eyes, and for pulling excess from the head, as in seizures.

BL 63 *Location:* Run your finger along the outside of the foot from the heel until you come to the bony bump. This point is where your finger stops just in front the bone.

Function: A good point for relieving pain and pulling excess from the head, as in seizures.

Kidney

KI 1 *Location:* In the "dent" below the toes when you curl up your foot; approximately a third of the distance between the toes and the heal.

Function: This is the first point of the Kidney channel, the lowest point on the body, a powerful point for calming the mind and the spirit and reviving consciousness.

KI 3   *Location:* In the hollow between the inside ankle and the Achilles tendon.

Function: The strongest and most versatile point on the Kidney channel. It is used for a variety of Kidney and Bladder conditions as well as for overall strengthening of other organs and the body as a whole.

KI 4   *Location:* First locate KI 3, then go approximately ½ FB below and ½ FB toward the Achilles tendon.

Function: This point can help stabilize emotions, such as fear associated with anorexia.

KI 6   *Location:* In the hollow directly below the inside anklebone.

Function: This is a strong point for activating Kidney energy, for treating insomnia (closes eyes).

KI 7   *Location:* First find KI 3, then come up the leg 2 FB above KI 3.

Function: This is a strong point for treating Kidney problems and edema.

Pericardium/Master of the Heart

P 5   *Location:* On the palm side of the forearm, 3 FB above the crease in the middle of the arm.

Function: Calms the spirit.

P 6   *Location:* On the palm side of the forearm, 2 FB above the crease in the middle of the arm.

Function: This is a major point that has many important uses. It opens the chest, and it can balance the body's Yin and Yang. It helps to calm the Heart, especially when a person is upset from a relationship.

Triple Burner

TB 3   *Location:* On the back of the hand, feel between the fourth and the little finger toward the wrist and you'll feel a "dent" before coming to a "bump."

     Function: This point is good for pain with bending fingers.

TB 4   *Location:* In the wrist crease on the back of the hand, below the fourth finger.

     Function: A good point for wrist pain.

TB 5   *Location:* On the back side of the forearm, 2 FB above the crease in the middle of the arm.

     Function: An important point for opening up channels, for balancing the Yin and Yang energies of the body, and for treating headache, especially when used with GB 41.

TB 8   *Location:* Start at the wristbone on the side of the fifth (little) finger and slide your finger along the middle edge of the bone up toward the elbow in the groove between two bones of the forearm. This point is located 4 FB above the wrist.

     Function: This is the crossing point for the three Yang channels of the arm: Large Intestine, Triple Burner, and Small Intestine. It can be used to activate energy movement across several parts of the body as well as to relieve pain in the arm.

TB 14 *Location:* Raise your arm to the side, to shoulder level. Find LI 15, then slide your finger along the shoulder toward the back. You'll feel a hollow on the side of the tip of the shoulderbone (acromion). In most people you can see a dimple or a depression there.

Functions: This is a very good point for treating shoulder pain, stiffness, weakness, shoulder injuries, or difficulty in raising the arm. Usually it is massaged along with LI 15 for local shoulder treatment.

TB 17 *Location:* Fold the earlobe forward, and the point is directly behind the earlobe in a hollow space next to the jawbone.

Function: A good point for treating ear problems.

TB 21 *Location:* Open the mouth and feel the point at the top of the tip of the jawbone right in front of the ear.

Function: A good point for treating a variety of ear problems. Often used with SI 19 and GB 2.

Gallbladder

GB 1 *Location:* In the hollow space next to the side corner of the eye.

Function: A good point for treating eye problems.

GB 2 *Location:* Open the mouth and feel the point at the bottom of the tip of the jawbone right in front of the ear.

Function: A good point for treating a variety of ear problems. Often used with TB 21 and SI 19.

GB 8 *Location:* Fold the ear to find the apex or the top point of the ear. This point is 1 FB above the apex.

Function: A good point for treating alcoholic intoxication.

GB 20 *Location:* Feel along the base of the skull. This point is usually the most tender spot in that area.

Function: This is an important point for treating "wind" conditions, headaches, and neck pain.

GB 21 *Location:* The highest point on the shoulder. Usually it is tender.

Function: This is a good point for shoulder pain.

GB 24 *Location:* Three rib spaces directly below the nipple

Function: This point is effective for sadness and sighing.

GB 29 *Location:* This point is difficult to locate, but is best found by lying on the side opposite the hip that hurts and feeling the top of your upper leg that is connected to the hipbone—the greater trochanter. You can locate it more easily by rotating your foot back and forth. Slide your finger slightly forward toward the groin. This point would be tender if you have hip pain. It is a deep point, so you need to apply firm massage.

Function: An excellent point for hip pain that goes to the groin area.

GB 30 *Location:* This point would be best located by lying on the side opposite the hip that hurts and bending the leg of the painful hip. Rotate your foot to locate the greater trochanter, as in GB 29; now move your finger back around the trochanter toward the buttock and slightly upward, toward the hip. It is approximately a third of the distance from the trochanter, in a line connecting the sacrum to the trochanter. It is a very deep point, so apply very firm massage.

Function: This is the "big point" for hip problems, for sciatica pain.

GB 31 *Location:* When you stand up, put your hands by your side and stretch out your fingers. The point is located right at the tip of your third finger.

Function: This point is good for pain on the side of the legs and for itching with urticaria.

GB 34 *Location:* Feel for the bottom of the kneecap; move your finger to the outside of the knee; feel the hollow or the space between the two bones.

Function: This is an important point for tendon and joint pains, as well as for pains along the side of the leg.

GB 40 *Location:* This point is located in the hollow space directly below and in front of the outside ankle.

Function: This point can help with spreading Liver Qi and make the joints less painful.

GB 41 *Location:* Move your finger from the web between the fourth and fifth toes up the foot. You'll feel a tendon. This point is on the *outside* (the side of the foot) of the tendon.

Function: A good point for treating headaches, especially when used with TB 5.

GB 43 *Location:* At the web between the fourth and the fifth toes.

Function: It is the water point on the GB channel and is good for treating headaches and swelling of the limbs.

GB 44 *Location:* Approximately 0.1 inch on the lower, outside corner of the fourth toe.

Function: A good distal point to clear the head and calm the spirit, as in restless insomnia with nightmares.

Liver

LR 1 *Location:* Right under the nail of the big toe on the side next to the second toe.

Function: Good for treating hangover, to retrieve consciousness, and to relieve drunkenness.

LR 2   *Location:* On the web between the first and the second toe, ½ FB up toward the foot.

Function: Fire point on the Liver channel. A good point for clearing Liver Fire; manifests as headaches or anger.

LR 3   *Location:* Run your finger from LR 2 in the inner space between the big and second toes toward the foot, 1½ FB from the edge of the web.

Function: On a par with LI 4 for importance in influencing the overall energy of the whole body, for general tonification (strengthening) of the body, and for calming the mind.

LR 5   *Location:* Five FB above the tip of the inside ankle bone, right behind the tibiabone.

Function: The LR channel goes to the throat and helps smooth Qi, as with excessive belching.

LR 8   *Location:* Bend your knee and put your finger on the inside knee crease. Then slide your finger straight up toward the top of the kneecap. This point is located in the big muscle mass between the crease and the top of the kneecap.

Function: This is the Water point of the Liver channel. It is used to tonify (strengthen) the Liver organ or channel. It also can be used for knee pain.

Conception Vessel—Major Yin Channel on Front of Body

CV 3   *Location:* One FB above the pubis in the midline.

Function: This is an important point for treating bladder disorders.

CV 4   *Location:* Two FB above the pubis in the midline.

Function: This is a very powerful point that can nourish the Kidney, Spleen, Small Intestine, and Lower Burner.

CV 5   *Location:* Three FB above the pubis in the midline.

Function: This regulates the three burners and fluid balance in the body.

CV 6   *Location:* One and one-half FB below the navel in the midline.

Function: Also known as "Dantian," the important and powerful Qi point mentioned in chapter 5 for Qigong. This is a very important point for tonifying and regulating Qi, is the master point for the Lower Burner, and also strengthens Kidney.

CV 7   *Location:* One FB below the navel in the midline.

Function: This is a good point for regulating menstruation and for strengthening the lower abdomen.

CV 8   *Location:* The belly button. This point is uncomfortable to massage.

Function: Important point for warming abdomen for any cold conditions by applying slices of warmed ginger or warming herbs.

CV 9   *Location:* One FB above the belly button.

Function: This is called the "water divide" point, which is good for "water diseases" such as ascites (fluid in the abdomen), or edema in the body, or vomiting after eating.

CV 10   *Location:* Two FB above the belly button.

Function: This point helps to decrease food stagnation and abdominal fullness and to regulate Stomach Qi.

CV 12   *Location:* Midway between the sternum and the navel.

Function: This is the master point for the Middle Burner

and is very powerful for digestive problems and for Stomach problems.

CV 15 *Location:* Right below the tip of the sternum, the bone that comes to the point in the middle of the chest.

Function: This point can regulate Heart Qi.

CV 17 *Location:* Between the nipples in the middle of the chest.

Function: This is a very important point for regulating and strengthening overall Qi and for strengthening the Lung and the Stomach.

CV 22 *Location:* This is the point right at the base of the neck in the front, above the breastplate bone.

Function: This is a good point for treating throat and voice problems and for treating cough.

CV 23 *Location:* In the midline of the throat, right above the Adam's apple.

Function: This point is useful for problems of the tongue and mouth.

Governing Vessel—Major Yang Channel on Midline of Back (DU)

DU 4 (Mingmen)   *Location:* First find BL 23. DU 4 is between the two BL 23 points on the spine.

Function: This is one of the most important points in the body. It is the famous Mingmen (Gate of Life) point. It is the root of life, of Yin and Yang.

DU 14 *Location:* See the discussion on Bladder Shu points to find C 7 vertebrae. DU 14 is directly below C 7 in the midline of the spine.

Function: This is an important point for treating fever and wind syndromes.

DU 16 *Location:* Feel with your thumb or finger along the midline of the back of the head. This point is immediately below the "bump" at the base of the skull.

Function: This point is the "palace of wind" that can harmonize Qi flow to the brain, especially in wind conditions, in external wind conditions and in internal wind conditions such as seizures.

DU 20 *Location:* Fold the ears and find the apex or the top point. Put your thumbs on the two apices and bring your third fingers touching at the middle of the head. DU 20 is located at the intersection between a line drawn in the middle of the face from the tip of the nose with the line drawn from the top of the ears. This is the location of the crown of the head.

Function: This is a very important and powerful point. It is known as BaHui, the Hundred Meeting Place, and is the intersection of all the Yang energies. It is also the point for bringing in Qi from Heaven during Qigong exercises.

DU 22 *Location:* At the top of the head, 2 FB behind the hairline in the midline.

Function: For hangover headache with excessive alcohol.

DU 26 *Location:* Above the upper lip, in the midline, two-third distance from the upper lip, one-third distance from the base of the nose.

Function: This is an emergency point for treating loss of consciousness and acute seizures.

Extra Points

Anmian *Location:* This point is located behind the ear.

Function: The name means "Peaceful Sleep" and is used to treat insomnia.

Ding Chuan   *Location:* First find DU 14. Ding chuan points are located ½ FB to the side of the DU 14 on both sides.

Function: The name means "Stop Wheeze" and is used to treat acute asthma.

Yintang (third eye)   *Location:* In the midpoint between the middle edges of eyebrows.

Function: This is a very important calming point.

Taiyang   *Location:* In the "dent" in the temporal area, approximately 1 FB from the outside corner of the eye.

Function: This is a good point for treating headaches.

MN-LE 16   *Location:* This is the inside "eye" of the knee, with ST 35 as the outside "eye" of the knee.

Function: This is one of the points for treating knee pain, weakness of the knee.

M-UE 29   *Location:* Two points located 4 FB above the middle of the wrist crease on the palm side, one on each side of the tendon. Can massage with a back-and-forth motion with the thumb across the arm.

Function: To treat hemorrhoids.

Ba Xie   *Location:* Make the hand into a fist. The points are in the web spaces closer to the fingers.

Function: Good points for treating finger pain and stiffness.

Lao Gong   *Location:* Make a fist with your fingers. The point in the palm of the hand between the tip of the middle and the fourth (ring) finger is the Lao Gong point.

Function: This is translated as "Hard Working" point. It is used in Qigong to activate Qi. It also corresponds to the abdomen on the hand microsystem.

Mingmen   See DU 4.

LUNG MERIDIAN

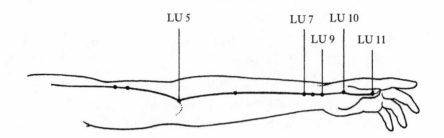

LU 5   LU 7   LU 10

LU 9   LU 11

LARGE INTESTINE MERIDIAN

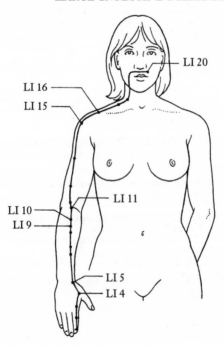

LI 20

LI 16

LI 15

LI 11

LI 10

LI 9

LI 5

LI 4

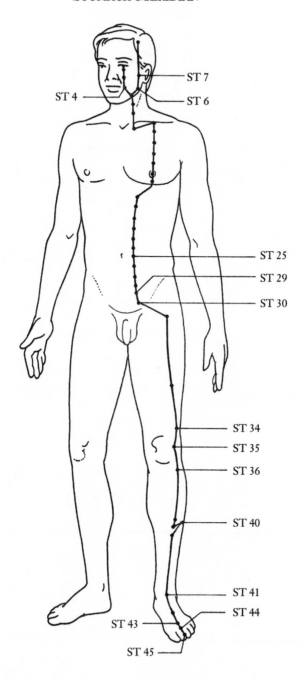

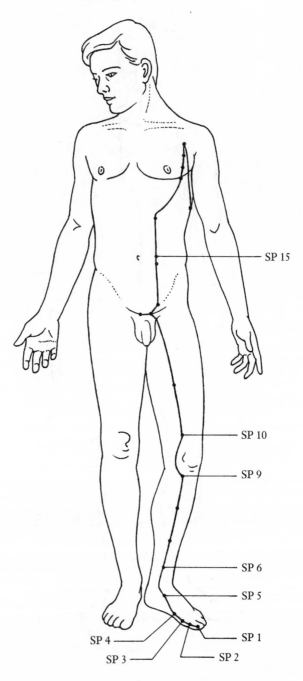

SP 15

SP 10

SP 9

SP 6

SP 5

SP 4

SP 1

SP 3

SP 2

HEART MERIDIAN

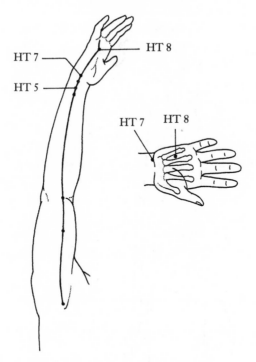

HT 7

HT 8

HT 5

HT 7   HT 8

SMALL INTESTINE MERIDIAN

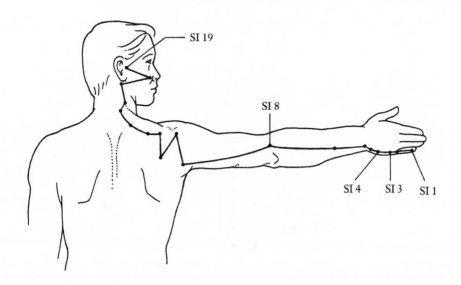

SI 19

SI 8

SI 4   SI 3   SI 1

BLADDER MERIDIAN

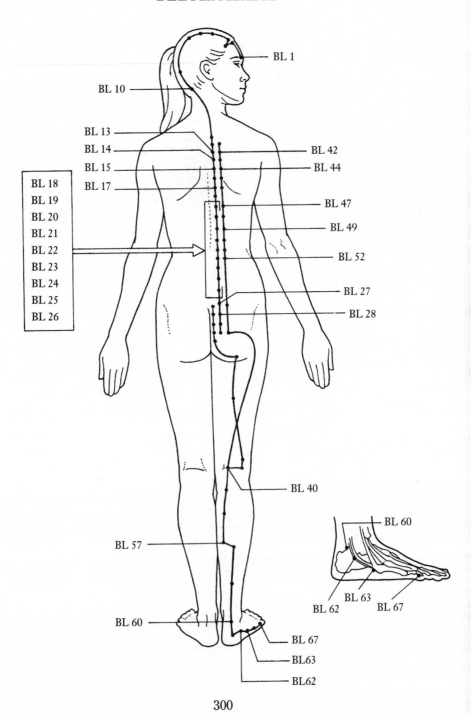

BL 1

BL 10

BL 13
BL 14
BL 15
BL 17

BL 42
BL 44

BL 47

BL 49

BL 52

BL 27

BL 28

BL 18
BL 19
BL 20
BL 21
BL 22
BL 23
BL 24
BL 25
BL 26

BL 40

BL 60

BL 57

BL 63

BL 62

BL 67

BL 60

BL 63

BL 62

BL 67

300

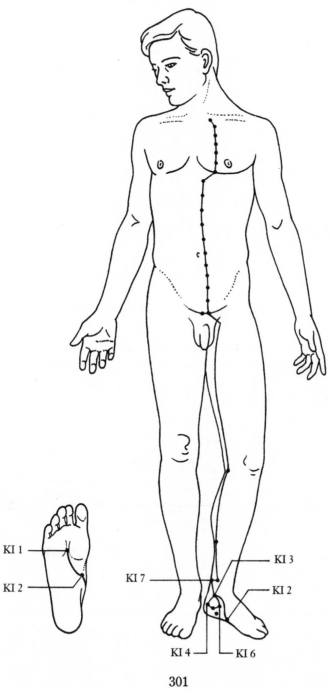

KI 1

KI 2

KI 3

KI 7

KI 2

KI 4   KI 6

PERICARDIUM MERIDIAN

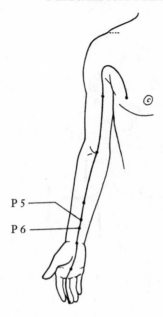

P 5 —
P 6 —

TRIPLE BURNER MERIDIAN

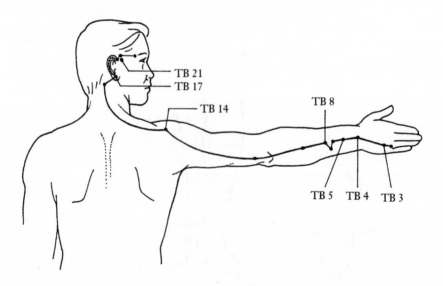

TB 21
TB 17
TB 14
TB 8
TB 5   TB 4   TB 3

GALLBLADDER MERIDIAN

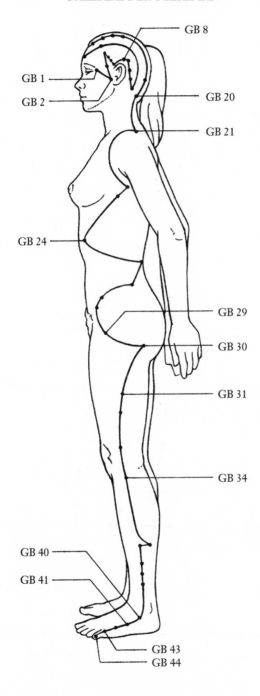

GB 8

GB 1

GB 2

GB 20

GB 21

GB 24

GB 29

GB 30

GB 31

GB 34

GB 40

GB 41

GB 43
GB 44

LIVER MERIDIAN

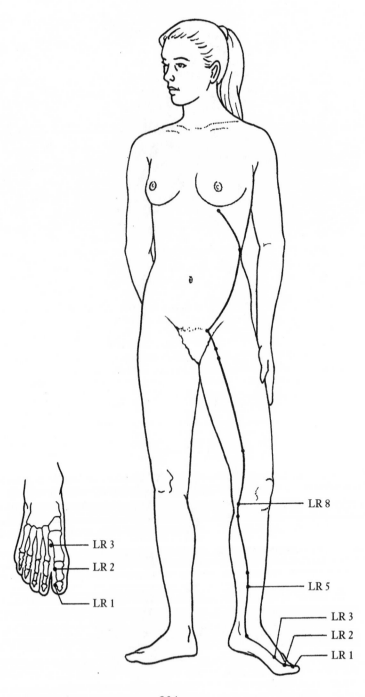

LR 8

LR 5

LR 3
LR 2
LR 1

LR 3
LR 2
LR 1

CONCEPTION VESSEL MERIDIAN

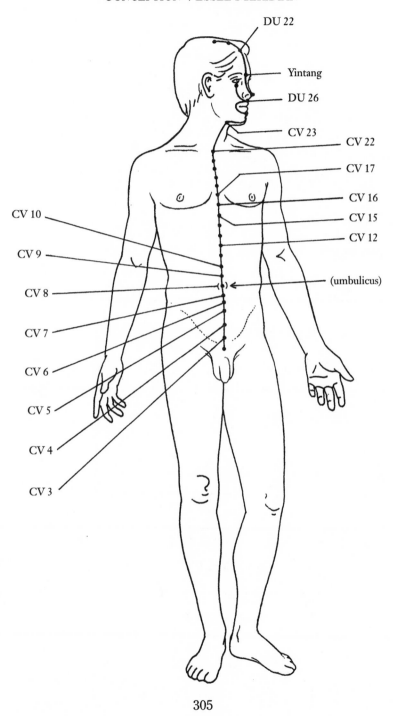

GOVERNING VESSEL MERIDIAN

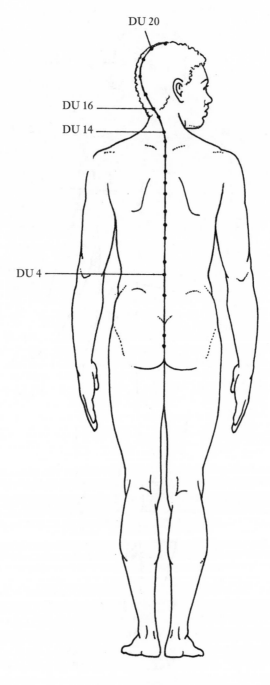

FRONT OF THE FACE

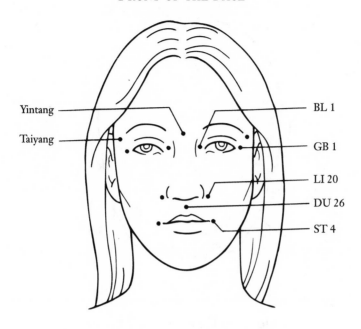

Yintang

BL 1

Taiyang

GB 1

LI 20

DU 26

ST 4

SIDE OF THE HEAD

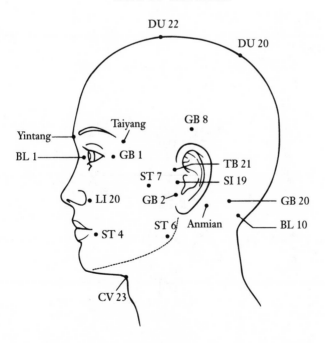

DU 22

DU 20

GB 8

Taiyang

Yintang

BL 1

GB 1

TB 21

ST 7

SI 19

LI 20

GB 2

GB 20

ST 4

ST 6

Anmian

BL 10

CV 23

TOP OF THE HEAD

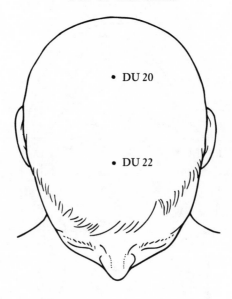

• DU 20

• DU 22

OUTSIDE VIEW OF LOWER ARM

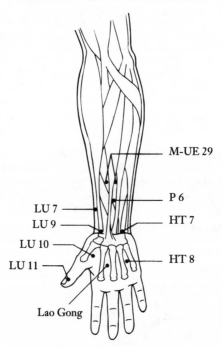

M-UE 29

P 6

LU 7

LU 9

HT 7

LU 10

LU 11

HT 8

Lao Gong

OUTSIDE VIEW OF ARM

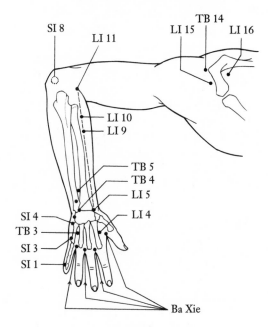

SIDE VIEW OF LOWER ARM

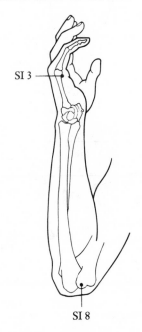

FRONT VIEW OF LOWER LEG

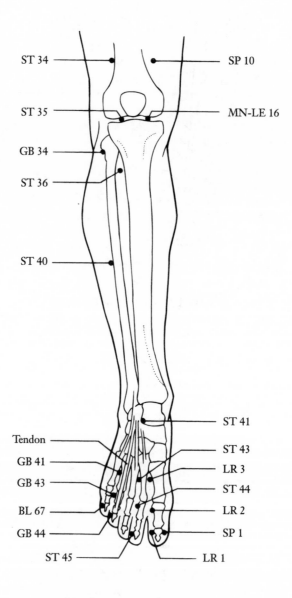

ST 34   SP 10

ST 35   MN-LE 16

GB 34

ST 36

ST 40

                 ST 41

Tendon   ST 43

GB 41   LR 3

GB 43   ST 44

BL 67   LR 2

GB 44   SP 1

ST 45   LR 1

Inside View of Lower Leg

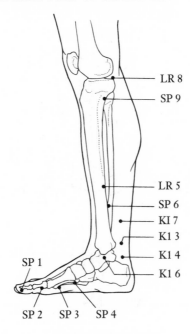

LR 8
SP 9
LR 5
SP 6
KI 7
K1 3
K1 4
K1 6
SP 1
SP 2   SP 3   SP 4

Outside View of Lower Leg

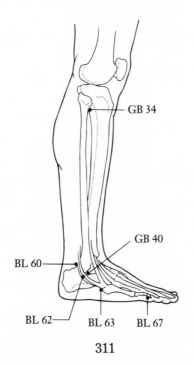

GB 34
GB 40
BL 60
BL 62   BL 63   BL 67

BACK OF THE HAND MICROMERIDIANS

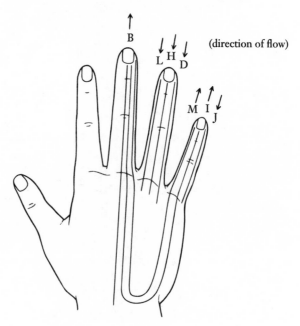

(direction of flow)

PALM-SIDE MICROMERIDIANS

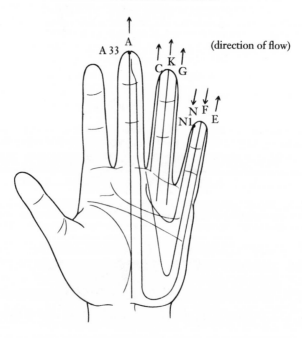

(direction of flow)

Palm Correspondence Chart

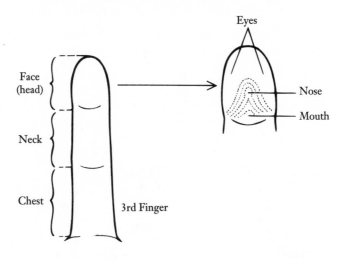

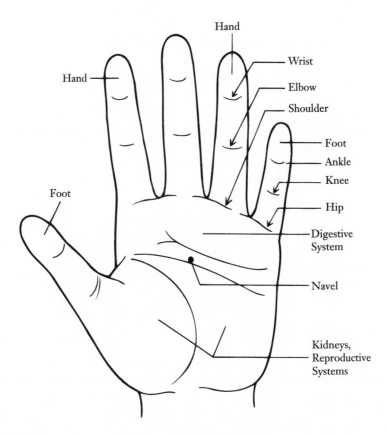

313

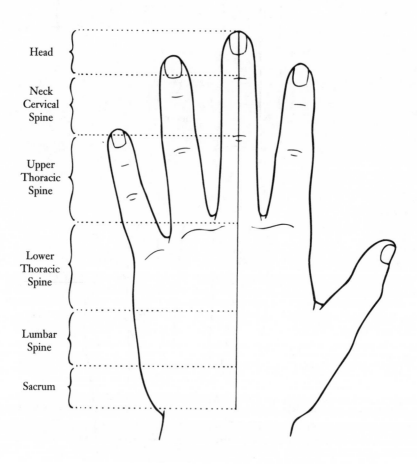

Bibliography

Adams, R. D., and Victor, M. *Principles of Neurology.* New York: McGraw-Hill, 1993.

Baldry, P. E. *Acupuncture, Trigger Points, and Musculoskeletal Pain.* London: Churchill Livingstone, 1993.

Barkely, R. A. *Attention-Deficit Hyperactivity Disorder: A Handbook for Diagnosis and Treatment.* New York: Guilford Press, 1998.

Becker, R. *Cross Currents: The Perils of Electropollution, the Promise of Electromedicine.* New York: G. P. Putnam's Sons, 1990.

Beinfield, H., and Korngold, E. *Between Heaven and Earth: A Guide to Chinese Medicine.* New York, Ballantine Books, 1991.

Bensky, D., and Gamble A., trans. and comp. *Materia Medica: Chinese Herbal Medicine.* Seattle: Eastland Press, 1993.

Cao, J., et al. *Essentials of Traditional Chinese Pediatrics.* Beijing: Foreign Language Press, 1990.

Chang, C. C. *Shang Han Lun: Wellspring of Chinese Medicine,* ed. Hong-Yen Hsu and William G. Peacher, Long Beach, Calif: Keats, 1981.

China Zhenjiuology: A Series of Teaching Videotapes. Chinese Medical Audio-Video Organization/Meditalent Enterprises, 1990s.

Chow E. P. Y. Personal instructions and communication.

Chow, E. P. Y., and McGee, C. T. *Miracle Healing from China . . . Qigong.* Coeur D'Alene, Idaho: Medipress, 1996.

Deadman, P., and Al-Kahafaji, M. *A Manual of Acupuncture.* East Sussex, Eng.: *Journal of Chinese Medicine Publications,* 1998.

"Diagnosis and Treatment of Gynecology and Pediatrics." In *Chinese Zhenjiuology: A Series of Teaching Videotapes.* Chinese Medical Audio-Video Organization/Meditalent Enterprises, 1990s.

Ellis, A. Personal communication.

Ellis, E.; Wiseman, N.; and Boss K. *Fundamentals of Chinese Acupuncture,* rev. ed. Brookline, Mass: Paradigm, 1991.

Encyclopaedia Britannica. CD-ROM, 1998.

English-Chinese Encyclopedia of Practical Traditional Chinese Medicine. Vols. 1–14. Beijing: Higher Education Press, 1990.

Fan, Y. L. *Chinese Pediatric Massage Therapy: A Parent's and Practitioner's Guide to the Treatment and Prevention of Childhood Disease.* Boulder, Colo: Blue Poppy Press, 1994.

Fauci, A. S., et al., eds. *Harrison's Principles of Internal Medicine,* 14th ed. New York: McGraw-Hill, 1998.

Flaws, B. *A Handbook of TCM Pediatrics: A Practitioner's Guide to the Care and Treatment of Common Childhood Diseases.* Boulder, Colo.: Blue Poppy Press, 1997.

Gascoigne, S. *The Chinese Way to Health: A Self-Help Guide to Traditional Chinese Medicine.* Boston, Charles E. Tuttle, 1997.

Helms, J. *Acupuncture Energetics: A Clinical Approach for Physicians.* Berkeley, Calif.: Medical Acupuncture, 1995.

Hoeprich, P. D.; Jordan, M. C.; and Ronald, A. R., eds. *Infectious Diseases: A Treatise of Infectious Processes.* Philadelphia: J. B. Lippincott, 1994.

Loo, M. "Alternative Therapies in Children." In *Complementary/Alternative Medicine: An Evidence-Based Approach,* edited by J. W. Spencer and J. Jacobs. St. Louis: Mosby, 1999.

Lu, H. *Chinese Foods for Longevity: The Art of Long Life.* New York: Sterling, 1990.

Maciocia, G. *The Foundations of Chinese Medicine: A Comprehensive Text for Acupuncturists and Herbalists.* London: Churchill Livingstone, 1989.

———. *Obstetrics and Gynecology in Chinese Medicine.* New York: Churchill Livingston, 1998.

———. *The Practice of Chinese Medicine: The Treatment of Diseases with Acupuncture and Chinese Herbs.* London: Churchill Livingstone, 1994.

———. *Tongue Diagnosis in Chinese Medicine.* Seattle: Eastland Press, 1995.

Matsumoto, K., and Birch, S. *Five Elements and Ten Stems: Nan Ching Theory, Diagnostics, and Practice.* Brookline, Mass: Paradigm, 1983.

Microsoft Encarta Encyclopedia. CD-ROM, 1998.

Mussat, Maurice. *"Acupuncture Energetic Lectures."* Videotape. Los Angeles: UCLA.

Nei Ching: The Yellow Emperor's Classic Internal Medicine, trans. Ilza Veith. Berkeley: University of California Press, 1949.

Nelson, W. E., et al., eds. *Nelson's Textbook of Pediatrics,* 15th ed. Philadelphia: W. B. Saunders, 1996.

Ni, M., and McNease, C. *The Tao of Nutrition.* Santa Monica, Calif.: SevenStar Communications, 1987.

O'Connor, J., and Bensky, D., eds. *Acupuncture: A Comprehensive Text.* Seattle: Eastland Press, 1981.

Oleson, T. *Auriculotherapy Manual: Chinese and Western Systems of Ear Acupuncture.* Los Angeles: Health Care Alternatives, 1996.

Palmer, M. *The Elements of Tao.* Rockport, Mass: Elements, 1991.

Physicians' Desk Reference. Oradell, N.J.: Medical Economics, 1999.

Physicians' Desk Reference for Nonprescription Drugs. Montvale, N.J.: Medical Economics Data Production, 1999.

Pitchford, P. *Healing with Whole Foods: Oriental Traditions and Modern Nutrition*. Berkeley, Calif.: North Atlantic Books, 1993.

Raquena, Y. *Terrains and Pathology in Acupuncture. Vol. I, Correlations with Diathetic Medicine*. Brookline, Mass.: Paradigm, 1986.

Reid, D. *The Complete Book of Chinese Health and Healing: Guarding the Three Treasures*. Boston: Shambhala, 1995.

Rosenberg, Z. Lectures and personal communication, 1999.

Schuller, D. E., and Schleuning, A. J. II. *DeWeese and Saunders' Otolaryngology: Head and Neck Surgery*. St. Louis: Mosby, 1994.

Scott, J. *Acupuncture in the Treatment of Children*. London: Eastland Press, 1991.

Shanghai Xin-Hua Hospital. Personal observations, 1999.

Sleisenger, M. H., and Fordtran, J. S., eds. *Gastrointestinal Disease*. Vols. I and II, *Pathophysiology/Diagnosis/Management*. Philadelphia. W.B. Saunders, 1993.

Spencer, J. W., and Jacobs, J., eds. *Complementary/Alternative Medicine: An Evidence-Based Approach*. St. Louis: Mosby, 1999.

Thurston, W. B. Personal communication, 1999.

Treatise on Febrile Diseases Caused by Cold with 500 Cases. Beijing, New World Press, 1993.

Yoo, T. W., *Koryo Hand Acupuncture*, Vol. I, Seoul: Eum Yang Mek Jin, 1977.

Yoo, T. W., et al; Lectures and personal communication, 1996–1998.

Zhu, Master. Personal instructions and communication, 1998, 1999.

———. *Qi Gong for Long Life*. HangZhou, China, 1999.

Index

319